PRAISE

"The perfect blend of entertainment and instruction."
~Erin Banco
International Journalist

"A fascinating story that will fill your heart with a passion for better health."   ~Michelle Stout
Brecknock, PA

"...valuable information that any person can use to improve their health...I couldn't put it down."
~ Michael P. Butterworth
MP Butterworth & Assoc.
Reading, PA

"... an inspiring, incredibly well-researched journey to a healthy lifestyle. Kate offers a solution to America's childhood obesity epidemic, and her Silent Cure teaches us that it is never too early or too late to begin a healthy nutrition/exercise program."
~Dan Batz
Pasadena Elite Fitness
Pasadena, CA

"Kate shares her very personal journey to a plant-based lifestyle in this hilariously funny, very honest, and eye-opening book. Sometimes I laughed, sometimes I cried, and sometimes I just poured myself a big glass of almond milk!"
~Rene Grove
Reading, PA

"...beautifully written, Kate Murray, a true health visionary seeks to educate people on cataclysmic health issues that rage against our country."
~Scott Einiger, Esq.
Abrams, Fensterman, Fensterman, Eisman,
Formato, Ferrara & Einiger, LLP
New York, NY

A Silent Cure
in my
Back Yard

*This book will shatter the foundation
of everything you once believed to be true
about proper nutrition.*

Disclaimer

The purpose of this book and the website, http://asilentcure.org is strictly to provide education, information, counseling, opinions and referrals. The author is not licensed to diagnose, prescribe or treat, but rather provide the reader with a general understanding of important issues related to health and disease.

By using my website and reading my book, you understand that there is no doctor-patient relationship between you, A Silent Cure, Vogue Media and/or its affiliates. The information offered should not be used as a substitute for competent medical advice from a licensed professional physician. The information is educational in nature and should not be regarded as a recommendation for self-medication in the absence of proper medical supervision.

A Silent Cure and/or Vogue Media is not responsible for any direct, indirect, incidental, consequential or any other damages arising in connection with the services and information provided. You agree to defend, indemnify, and hold A Silent Cure, Vogue Media, Kate Murray, its officers, directors, employees, agents, and certified educators harmless from and against any claims, actions or demands, liabilities and settlements including without limitation, reasonable legal and accounting fees, resulting from, or alleged to result from, your misunderstanding, misinterpretation, or misuse of the aforementioned conditions.

Additional Notes: The charts and recipes referenced herein are not available in the e-version of this book, they are only available in the paperback version.

ACKNOWLEDGEMENTS

For my husband, Steve, your endearing support and resolve have enabled us to build a strong foundation for our children. Thank you for continuously eating strange plants that you've never heard of, and for putting up with my sharp and candid point of view.

To my Dad, Lou, it is your wisdom that inspires me to keep reaching higher, and continuously challenges me to seek out answers. Your example has always encouraged me to strive for the perfect balance. Thank you, the world over, for everything you do for me and my family. And for my mom: whose guiding spirit shines down from heaven influencing each decision I make. I miss you with all my heart.

Ann and Louis: The two people in this world who are most like me. Thank God someone understands that life is not always about the destination. I love you guys.

Kim, Valerie, and Kent: Thank you for allowing me many opportunities to experiment with new recipes. This book would not have been possible if it weren't for your commitment to making sure my kids had something to do; it means so much to me.

Erin and Sarah: It isn't often you find family comprised of women who are also truly great friends. Technology today has enabled us to stay in touch with one another in a way our parents could never have envisioned. Many thanks to you for coming along on this journey with me.

Lisa: My editor and personal therapist. Thank you for all of your inspiration and your candidly objective point of view. Your recommendations have been invaluable. I couldn't have done this without you.

Michelle: My personal cheerleader...there is a reason for everything in this life. I believe that Kylie will have a happier, healthier future because of your commitment to your health. I'm truly grateful for all of your suggestions along the way.

To all of my dear friends who shared their own most personal stories: Thank you for providing a first-hand account of the trials and tribulations involved in your own personal lives, and the lives of your families. Because of the challenges you shared, I think I have been able to help my readers understand how they too can become empowered by the knowledge that they truly can gain control of a disease that may have otherwise destroyed their life. You already know that life's greatest reward is always at the end of a journey of hard work, dedication, and motivation. You were willing to take the risks to get there. For that, you are to be commended. I'm not going to name any names here because there are so many, but please know that I know who you are, and I thank each and every one of you, for all of our conversations.

Forward

by: Erin Banco

I grew up in a family that loved to eat. During the holidays, we would sit at the dinner table for hours, filling our plates with first helpings, second helpings, and sometimes even third helpings. We would talk for hours over our indulging. Then we would nap, and return to the kitchen for the next meal. It was bliss. But it was not only the act of eating that I came to love—it was what was on my plate.

Over the years, I developed a love of food. I love everything about it. From where it is grown, to where it is sold, to how it tastes. Now, as an adult, I have translated that love of food into a passion for cooking. For a while, I held onto my roots. I didn't stray too far from the diet I had as a child (pasta, potatoes, and red meat). But that diet quickly changed when I took a job overseas.

When I came home, I couldn't wait to start cooking again. But my appetite was different, and the conversation about food had changed. My friends were dieting, or had turned vegan. Everyone seemed to be interested in eating a strictly plant-based diet. I had no idea what that meant, or why it mattered, until I read A Silent Cure in my Back Yard.

For the average American, a usual day consists of going to work, paying the bills, and putting food on the table for the family. Our days become consumed with other priorities, and food is the last thing on our minds. Many of us have resorted to Lean Cuisine or fast food restaurants. I have fallen into this category many times.

This book motivated me to think more about the food I am eating and what affect it will have on my body. After I came back to the U.S. from traveling, I had lost more than ten pounds, and I was looking to regain some of my strength. But I had cut out meat from my diet, and I couldn't figure out how to cook meals for myself that would give me enough protein and calories to make me feel better. I did not have time to take courses or to self educate myself on how to eat healthier. A Silent Cure in my Back Yard was the key. Murray was my navigator. The book was both a coach and an encourager.

Did you ever wonder what the certifications on the front of cereal boxes meant? Do you know how to read a nutrition label properly? Do you know why oil is bad for you? What about tiredness? Do you understand why you are tired almost everyday around 3 p.m.? Murray has all these answers and more in A Silent Cure in my Back Yard.

In her book, Murray laces together the perfect combination of personal storytelling with educational nutrition material. She lays out the most important information needed for the average American to understand why eating a plant-based diet matters, and provides the raw facts about how certain types of food affect our health. And I don't just mean that carrots make your eyesight better. Murray delves into the science of how different nutrients contribute to some of the most deadly diseases on the planet. But even with the scientific writing, Murray finds ways to keep the reader engaged; you will laugh, cry, and grit your teeth all in one sitting. Murray's dedication for her work comes from a place of both sorrow and joy. Her words will warm your heart, and make you rethink all of the lessons you were taught about healthy eating. A Silent Cure in my Backyard is the perfect blend of entertainment and instruction.

Murray examines the why. She looks at the reasons why we should consider eating healthier and following a plant-based diet. She forces the reader to contemplate how their day-to-day lives might be different if they paid more attention to the food they eat. This book can be understood and enjoyed by every kind of person that picks it up. Whether you are a college student on a budget, a runner looking to eat right, or a mother who wants to experiment with plant-based cooking—A Silent Cure in my Back Yard is for all of us.

~*Erin Banco, International Journalist*

TABLE OF CONTENTS

Part III

The Rise of the Organic Generation

Part IV

Scientifically Speaking

Part V
The Cancer Mantra

Part VI
Motivation: Celebrate the Delectable Plant

Part V: Resources

For Carla and Joe:
May you have the courage
to lead a life of happiness and balance.

A Silent Cure
in my
Back Yard

INTRODUCTION

Before people can truly understand kindness and compassion, they have to know sorrow. I believe there are certain things a person has to live through in order to gain a real appreciation for life. One of them is watching someone die. Whether it is witnessing a terrifying car accident first hand, seeing a runner collapse at mile 18, or acting as a caregiver for someone with a debilitating or terminal illness, the intense emotion evoked by that experience will change a person forever.

My outlook changed. My approach changed. I suddenly became hypersensitive about everything from preserving pictures, video, and family traditions to cursing anyone who drifted through a stop sign or drove diagonally across painted parking spaces. It occurred to me that this life we have is precious, and if there is something we can do to protect ourselves from illness, then why isn't everyone doing it? The short answer is that people either haven't been personally touched by disease, or they just don't realize how much control we really do have over many illnesses, including not only vascular diseases and cancer, but chronic, auto-immune diseases as well.

…PEOPLE EITHER HAVEN'T BEEN

PERSONALLY TOUCHED BY IT,

OR THEY DON'T REALIZE

HOW MUCH CONTROL WE REALLY DO HAVE

OVER MANY ILLNESSES…

Before you is an epic narration of courage, small triumphs, and ultimately defeat; it is a familiar story for many people, and it's becoming all too familiar for many more.

My mom died of cancer when my son was 2 weeks old, it was a confluence of miracle and loss. My emotions were already in need of repair after pregnancy and childbirth, so my desire for a ritual to help sort through the sadness was intense. I couldn't spend my life wallowing in sorrow about missing my mom because how would I care for my children? Running outdoors through the natural elements, the sun, wind, and rain, became my inner peace. Exactly six weeks after my second C-section, I found my way back to running; I ran 26.2 miles to honor the memory of my mother. Over the past few years, everyone from new moms to seasoned athletes has asked me how I managed marathon training with two young children, less than 14 months apart. The truth is, I found an inner contentment, a sense of calmness within my own heart; instead of placing blame on something or someone else for the loss and heartache, I learned to find answers in my own motivations.

As the story unfolds, it no longer became a marathon to honor my mom, it was a way to connect her memories to my life and to the lives of my children whom she would never know. For every mile, every 3 hour long training run, every time I got out there and ran through the rain, the snow, and the "I wish I was still sleeping in my warm bed" syndrome, it was all the beginning of my own purpose. Whenever I experienced any kind of pain, I knew in my heart it wasn't nearly as difficult as what she went through each day just to live in this world.

Her battle with breast cancer, then ultimately leukemia wasn't supposed to happen. It wasn't genetic or an inherited disease; in 2001 she was diagnosed with Breast Cancer, and within a month, underwent chemotherapy, then the mastectomy. She was blessed to be considered among those who had beat the cancer...or so we thought. Then, in 2006, within an instant it seemed, she was diagnosed with a condition called Acute Myeloid Leukemia (AML), a rapidly spreading blood cancer, that was brought about by the chemotherapy she received during her treatments for breast cancer...5 years prior.

At the time, my parents strategically followed the advice of the medical professionals, and my mom fought hard, like millions of people do, until the bitter end. She was the strongest person I've ever known. Every value she stood for is a legacy I hope my children will come to understand some day.

The top 5 types of cancer in the United States according to the American Cancer Society's 2011 Report[4] (the most current available as of this writing) are Lung, Breast & Prostate, Colon & Rectum, and Pancreatic cancer. It is estimated that over 240,000 people will be diagnosed with breast cancer alone this year.

ONLY BETWEEN 5 AND 10%
OF ALL CANCERS IN THE UNITED STATES
ARE HEREDITARY.

It may surprise you that only between 5 and 10% of all cancers in the United States are hereditary.[5] Hmm. So if that is 240,000 people who died of cancer and only 24,000 of those cases were genetic, then what about the other 216,000 people who died of cancer last year? Where did the cancer inside their bodies come from?

Two Hundred and Sixteen Thousand people.

So, the "war on cancer" has claimed the lives of more Americans in one year than all the U.S. Military Wars combined.[38]

Before you assume you are susceptible to getting breast cancer because it runs in your family, first consider what you eat and whether it is similar to what your mother, grandmother, sister, or aunt ate throughout her lifetime. This is important, so listen up:

In the chapters that follow, I explain in excruciating detail, a very personal account of how I uncovered these facts about nutrition and disease, and you will truly discover how this book will shatter the foundation of everything you once believed to be true about proper nutrition.

Because of my passion for running, and my motivation for doing everything I could to prevent and protect my own family from this horrible disease, I became focused on the vital connection between nutrition and human life. It's a connection that threatens the power and profits of the pharmaceutical industry, an industry that thrives on nutritional ignorance and deceptive marketing of its poisons to the uninformed masses.

I began, just as everyone else does, by reading all the latest books about proper nutrition and endurance training. It led me down a path of exploring counter intuitive factors, in other words, why things are not always what they seem.

4

If the research is solid, then why aren't our medical doctors more focused on educating us about how proper nutrition can prevent and reverse these deadly diseases?

As I was finishing up this book, a review was published critically evaluating the American Cancer Society's 2012 guidelines[6] which now urges doctors to speak to their patients about eating right and exercising. Over the last 5 years, hundreds of studies have shown that diet and exercise are closely associated with survival rate. So why are we still not listening? It's unfortunate that intuitively, people are drawn to quick, easy, or often lazy solutions which can ultimately lead to the opposite of what we imagine should be true. This is evident in many factors of life, not only nutrition or athletics, but personal happiness and well-being too. When a child struggles to find an answer, human instinct is to tell the child the answer. Yet providing guidance and encouragement would instead allow the child to work out the problem in his or her own way, which might be entirely different from the solution we, as adults, imagined.

IF YOU'RE ALWAYS RACING

TO THE NEXT MOMENT,

WHAT HAPPENS TO THE ONE YOU'RE IN?

Just like children need guidance and encouragement, so do we as adults. We are bombarded with health information from every form of media. When you wake up in the morning, the news report says a glass of wine a day is bad for you. When you watch the news that night, a glass of wine might actually be good for you.

I began this journey by seeking out answers so I could protect my own family from disease. Instead of racing to the next moment, I stopped for a pause. I think we forget to do that in our technologically advanced society today where everyone is rushed, overbooked, and over-committed. Throughout my journey, I raised my own awareness of a critical issue that has somehow managed to pass over our entire culture: we tend to choose the instinctive or obvious option, when doing the opposite may actually produce the desired effect. It's kind of like athletic training…sometimes it's better to rest your muscles with a day of recovery so they can perform better during the next difficult workout. If you don't rest, your fatigued muscles will not produce the desired result. The same advice goes for what you eat; it's time to take the advice of all moms and grandmoms to heart: eating more fresh fruits and vegetables really will save your life! But there's more…a lot more. As you will soon find out…there's a "Devil in the Milk [27]."

This book is for you and me. It's for my family and your family, our friends, our neighbors, and all the hard working, tax paying people of our country. It's for those of us who are saving for our children's college education while we're still paying off our own. It's for all the moms and dads, parents and grandparents, singles and students. It's for those of us who have been stricken by cancer or cardiovascular disease, or have a loved one that is dealing with the ramifications of such debilitating misery.

Maybe we were told that heart disease runs in our family, so we are at a greater risk. Maybe we are otherwise active and healthy, but we've been told that because of a family history of high blood cholesterol we will need to take medication for the rest of our lives. Maybe we have been told that we need a baseline mammogram at the age of 40, because breast cancer runs in our family. I'm going to show you why that is not true, and precisely how I arrived at that conclusion.

Often times, beliefs we have stick with us because they seem to make sense, but in reality, we simply learned them from our mother or grandmother, so we believe them in our adult lives. It's a common, misleading assumption that guides our decision making about what kind of food we put in our mouths.

You probably never thought about why folks in rural China are not dying of heart disease and cancer at the same alarming rate that regular folks in the United States are. Today we live in a different society than we did 50 years ago; we grew up going to dance class or baseball practice after school instead of cultivating the family garden. We bring goldfish crackers and pretzels to the game for our younger child, because we believe it's healthier than chips and cookies. We choose a low-fat, fruit flavored yogurt because we think it's healthier for our children to eat than a freeze pop, but in actuality, that very notion is what is making our society fatter and sicker than ever before.

If you think you are a healthy eater, but you don't quite understand why a freeze pop is better than a fruit flavored yogurt, then you're in the right place. I too thought that the better choice was the yogurt until I began my research. In fact, I didn't realize the extent the choices I made (as the primary grocery shopper in the household) influenced every facet of my life and my children's lives until I was knee deep in scientific literature. Let's face it; regular people don't comb scientific research journals. The purpose of this book is to give you the truth about the foods you think are healthy, and the motivation to make some changes.

We all know we can do a better job of passing over the drive through or lessening the amount of refined sugars in our diet, but what you may not know yet is quite surprising...that many of the products touted as healthy alternatives are even *worse for your health than you previously thought.*

I am one of those people that continually seeks out answers, and I don't stop until I have evaluated all the sides to every story. I want straight facts, not shenanigans. I didn't invent the research, I'm just presenting it to you in a way I wish it would have been given to me...straight up, easy to understand. That is the premise for this entire book, to speak in a language that we all understand. If you aren't entirely clear on what I'm talking about, then sit back and get comfortable, it's a fascinating ride. This is my story; it is very personal and the evidence is compelling.

May you be truly empowered by what you're about to read. It will profoundly change your life.

~ Kate Murray

PART I
THE HEALTH CRISIS:
HOW IT CAME TO THIS

Chapter I:
A Fundamental Understanding

As I lay in bed, I listen to the silence and look at the clock: 2:47 am. Why am I still awake? My mind doesn't stop wandering as I reflect on what could very well be the most enduring question of all time...why do some people die at the age of 57 while others live to be 100? And so it begins. I keep listening, to the rhythm of the rain, the tender sound of my husband breathing; I'm thinking about how deep the landscape shadows of my room become in the darkness.

It's a profound topic that spans generations, touches every society, race, gender and age group. Cancer. It's around every corner. Lately it seems to affect all of us whether we choose to admit it or not; we all know someone who has been diagnosed. For some of us though, it's more than just the disease that we hear about. It's near and dear, because this desolate disease has weakened our soul and profoundly changed our lives forever.

The twenty-first century has produced the fattest, sickest people America has ever known. According to the American Cancer Society's Facts and Figures report for 2012, approximately 577,190 Americans are expected to die of cancer, more than 1,500 people a day. Cancer is the second most common cause of death in the US, exceeded only by heart disease, accounting for nearly 1 of every 4 deaths.[1] It's a logical assumption that cancer will surpass heart disease as the number 1 killer within the next few years.

What mainstream Americans do not know yet is that there is a secret, and the evidence is captivating. The rest of this book will shock you. It's a story that has been growing for years and has been told by many accomplished scholars, both within the medical profession as well as the scientific research community. The answer to this worldwide dilemma of course is quite simple, yet it will take an entire book to explain. Why? People simply are not listening; that is, until they *choose* to listen. American society is a living metaphor; while other cultures look at Americans from the outside, third-party perspective, we continue to live our lives with convenience winning out over stark reality.

An often overlooked but very important connection to the entire dilemma is that people who are *not* overweight are dying of these same diseases. Seemingly no one is immune...or are we? The answer of course is yes, diseases of the heart, more correctly said: the vascular system, as well as the most common cancers...breast, prostate, pancreatic, colorectal are preventable and curable, even in the later stages of diagnosis.

Wait. Did I just say those diseases could be prevented and cured? Did you have to look back? You don't. I did say that heart disease is curable. Cancer is curable. Why hasn't your doctor told you this? Why hasn't the media told you this? Why are we still raising money for the largest organizations in the world to fund research on these diseases when the research and media keep telling us that we're just one more step closer to a cure?

Consider this: People who exercise regularly and eat a healthy diet are not supposed to be tired at 3:00 in the afternoon. Do you consider yourself healthy? (Okay, for the most part?) Are you busy running around, stressed out about work or finances, trying to fit everything in to your schedule (maybe even a few trips to the gym each week) but still constantly fatigued?

Maybe you're even fit and healthy. Maybe you do exercise regularly and eat right, but why then, if you're following the United States Department of Agriculture (USDA) recommendations for a healthy, low-fat diet along with moderate exercise are you *still* plagued by fatigue, or worse, one of the aforementioned diseases? This is but one of the reasons that moved me to write this book. I felt compelled to share the drama of how I arrived at the conclusions I have. I am not a medical doctor, I am not a professional research scientist, and I am not a celebrity. I am simply an educated, hardworking American who has a strong passion for finding the truth, and a burning hatred of mediocrity. I like answers that make sense, and I never settle for information that complicates rather than clarifies.

I'm still lying in my bed, and now its 3:07 am. I'm wondering why I'm still awake. Let's face it, people don't know this because interpreting standard deviation isn't exactly a recreational read. Even if they do understand the technical aspect of research studies, quantitative analysis was difficult enough to process the first time around, regular people don't want to go back there again. Instead, we watch the news and read the paper. We sometimes read blogs or check Facebook, and we scroll through Twitter to see the latest news at home and around the world. We are heavily reliant on technology and that's okay, but when you Google a phrase looking for answers...how can you be sure the information you're reading is credible? Of course, there are ways to evaluate credibility online, but just like an airline pilot cannot fly a plane solely on cruise control, we can't make informed decisions about our health by listening to only one point of view.

Perhaps our infatuation with visual images online takes over, so we try out a recipe because a colorful photo on Pinterest catches our eye; but how often do you truly evaluate the ingredients before you make it?

I look at the recipe, then I see that it includes milk or eggs. This is not clean eating. Why is someone using the term "clean" and including ingredients like dairy? Social media is an incredible means to creativity, what shocks me the most is the widespread misinterpretation of what clean, healthy eating really is. My goal is purely to educate you on how and why this matters...and include just a little humor about industry corruption along the way.

At no point in the last 35 years did the news media in any form (high definition, electronic, mobile, or otherwise) actually come out and tell us that a cure for cancer or heart disease already exists. Why? Why weren't we told about it? How did I not know about the information that would have been so critical to my own mother's livelihood? And if I didn't know, *how many other people don't know*? None of my friends know. My family doesn't know. My neighbors don't know, in fact, hundreds of millions of people *just don't know*. We are educated people. In fact, university educated people are taught to question and critically evaluate, to think about things that do not have concrete answers, even when there is a concrete answer.

HUNDREDS OF MILLIONS OF PEOPLE
JUST DON'T KNOW!

Telling you to eat more vegetables isn't exactly seductive, and in fact, it's not the only means to better health; but not to worry, in the chapters that follow I'm going to spell out everything you need to know.

Why me? Well, first of all the news isn't actually new. In fact, many people who are already aware of this have some strong reasons why the so called "elephant in the room" has not yet hit mainstream America.

14

What do I mean by "elephant in the room"? Well, this is the metaphor the scholars use to illustrate that the cure for cancer already exists, and it can be found, literally, in your own back yard. I'll show you the research in a way that we can all relate to instead of speaking in such highly technical terms that it becomes utterly confusing. I'll spell it out so that you don't miss the point. I'll speak in a language that everyone can understand so that you can share it with your family and friends, the people you care about most. I'll give it to you straight up, impartially and without bias...perhaps most importantly, with no personal investment in anything other than finding the truth.

THE RESEARCH

Knowledge wise, our society is certainly further along than we were in 1970, but the important disconnect is that 90% of the American population is unaware of how the funding of our research dollars is tainted. Ask those in the know, such as physicians and epidemiologists at leading healthcare facilities across the country, geneticists, pharmacologists, in fact, ask a cancer patient and you're likely to get the same answer. The fact is twofold, number one, we spend billions of dollars a year on this research which revolves around finding a cancer tumor and killing the tumor. It is a misleading and ineffective model because cancer is not the result of just one tumor, it is a disease that is interconnected to many systems in our bodies, and these treatments that our dollars fund, as most all cancer patients know, actually causes degeneration that is evident within many other bodily systems.

Our research dollars then, the dollars that hardworking American's donate by the millions to societies, foundations, walks, and causes, have been taken over by an industry that weeds through the science, cherry picks the findings, and reports what they deem appropriate; many times based on a business relationship. Wow, yes, I said that. You thought it, and I said it.

So why the confusion?

When research scientists conduct large-scale human surveys in an attempt to find correlation between nutrition and disease, it is difficult to control all of the variables, including the reality of what people eat, their daily habits and even their genetic makeup. Perhaps even more difficult for the public, is how to make sense out of the findings that are reported in the news. Every day it seems, the news is reporting on a new study. We live in a world where adversarialism and conflict are actually moral issues, without which society would remain stagnant; whether for the sake of good or ill, everyone has the right to dissent. This moral dilemma is precisely why we even have a need for clarification of this topic. It seems easy enough to be able to cut healthcare costs for an entire country overnight if the right people just understood the system doesn't it?

In the end, what you need to know here is that I have no ties toward any of the industries in question (research related, agricultural, medical, pharmaceutical, scientific, or political). Therefore my hope is merely that this book provides the gateway which just might help you and your family advance into a healthier, happier future.

So with that, let's talk about…

Chapter 2:

Healthcare in America
Diseases of Affluence and Poverty

Those millions of healthcare dollars American's spend each year on research and development, medicine, drugs, and surgeries are all in an effort to cure disease; these diseases are referred to, in some circles, as the "diseases of affluence" [2].

First and foremost, I think the word "affluent" needs to be properly defined for this context. When people hear the word affluent, they automatically associate that word with wealth. Think celebrity, elite athlete, politician, or other people who have topped the list of the most prosperous; when in fact, in this context, the term affluent is actually referring to all the people in the United States of America. That's right, you and me. Regular, working class people. Even people who receive food stamps fit into this "affluent" category. How so? Well, for one thing, in the United States if someone needs a meal, we have an abundance of programs, food banks, shelters, church organizations, subsidized school lunch programs and the like which means that anyone who *really* needs to eat certainly may. Our own government as well as a multitude of social service and charitable organizations across the nation work hard to ensure that children are not hungry and that people are not deprived of basic human needs. In fact, in the U.S., someone who needs medical attention cannot be turned away either.

The 2009-2011 report on the USDA's Food and Nutrition Accomplishments (the most current available as of the time of this writing) outlines that their most significant accomplishment of the last 3 years is the Supplemental Nutrition Assistance Program (SNAP). Read: "food stamps". One of the issues garnering attention then, is the distinction between "affluence" and "excess". Next let's define excess. In his book, *In Defense of Food* (Penguin Books, 2008), author Michael Pollan describes our nation as being "fatter and sicker" than ever before; in other words, implying a person could weigh 300 lbs. but still be *deficient* in the most essential nutrients of human life. Have you ever been standing in line at the grocery store and observed someone with a cart full of packaged food…paying with food stamps? Have you ever wondered why their cart is filled with kool-aid and pop tarts instead of apples, lettuce, and vegetables?

The common belief is that it costs a lot of money to eat healthy food, but in reality, it costs far less to fill up a cart with healthy food than it does to fill up a cart with packaged food. So why the misconception? What it comes down to is a matter of priority, and this is why we are a nation of excess. The economic downturn of the late 2000s definitely resulted in a substantial need for many American families; but perhaps the more striking issue though, is the fact that those hardworking Americans (who are ultimately paying for other people's food stamps) are the ones who are actually being taken advantage of by our own government. The term "affluent" is relative.

If a family collects government subsidized benefits because they cannot afford to buy healthy food, yet their windows are open wide enough that when I drive by, I can see a large screen television hanging on the wall, that is not in poverty, it is a matter of *priority*. Luxuries such as those are not essential to human life, they are *luxuries* and they cost money. What ends up happening with our current "system" is that the hardworking people fund those large screen .

televisions at the expense of quality food for the children of the families who really do need assistance.

Food is essential to human life. In other words, if you have the luxury of a roof over your head and something in your cabinet to eat when you're hungry, I am sorry to say that you are *not* living in poverty. If your house is in danger of being foreclosed upon but you watch television with a satellite dish, get regular manicures, and own a smartphone, you are *not* living in poverty; you simply need to get your priorities in order. If you live in a remote location of Ethiopia with merely a tent over your head and a scarcity of clean water to drink, *then* you are living in poverty. All cynicism aside, the aforementioned example is intended to distinguish between affluence and poverty, not point a stick in someone's eye for goodness sake. In a perfect world I would appreciate the luxury of getting my nails done on a regular basis too, but heck I need to make sure my kids eat first!

Okay, so basically we're all affluent in this context. The next important word to understand is excess. The instance of obesity in America is higher than in any other country in the world. *In the world.* The wealthiest nation in the world is eating itself to death. In other words, people who live in a remote locale like rural Ethiopia or China are not dying of the two most prevalent causes of death in the United States: heart disease and cancer (the diseases of affluence) instead they are dying of the diseases of "poverty" which are infectious diseases such as tuberculosis, meningitis, or diphtheria. These types of diseases are controllable in developed countries with proper medical attention.

Why does this discussion even matter? Well, if you think critically about this for just one moment, how can it be that in some parts of the world, people's lives are cut short by cancer and heart disease, and in other parts of the world, the instance of cancer and heart disease are practically non-existent?

"...HOW CAN IT BE THAT IN SOME PARTS OF THE WORLD, PEOPLE'S LIVES ARE CUT SHORT BY CANCER AND HEART DISEASE, AND IN OTHER PARTS OF THE WORLD, THE INSTANCE OF CANCER AND HEART DISEASE ARE PRACTICALLY NON-EXISTENT?"

This is the very question that scientific researchers have been measuring and evaluating with literally hundreds, possibly thousands of studies on longevity, disease and nutrition over the past 30 years. Therefore, it is critical to conclude the diseases of "affluence" are *very closely associated with the foods we eat.*

We have the ability to choose our foods in America, whether we choose cheese curls or grapes, whether we use our own hard earned money or government subsidized funds, whether we take the public transit to the grocery store or visit a soup kitchen, the reality is, most people in America *do* have access to food.

It's important to gain a fundamental understanding of how this problem, of Americans being fatter and more prone to disease than ever before in the history of the world, came to be. We already know the obvious... that fast food restaurants and packaged, processed foods are hard to come by in rural Ethiopia. Rather, even in remote villages of rural China for example, you may find a third-world marketplace where people still barter, trade, and sell what they grow themselves. What you haven't yet heard, what I'm just beginning to unlock for you, is perhaps the most shocking part of this whole story: understanding the dynamic of politics and science within the walls of some of the largest and most influential institutions of our society is of extreme importance to virtually everyone in America. In order to understand how to cure disease, you must first have a solid handle on understanding why disease is so prevalent in the first place.

Ah. Politics. At the root of every evil. What institutions am I talking about? Well, take the United States Department of Agriculture (USDA) for example; this institution issues the food guidelines that most American citizens follow...remember the food pyramid? I suppose if you're over 35 you do; in recent years the food pyramid has been replaced with the "My Plate" recommendation.[3] This is the guideline that schools, military personnel, hospitals and basically everyone is supposed to follow to be healthy. Those recommendations need to be much more specific. The guidelines go back to vague generalities such as "eat more vegetables and whole grains and eat less saturated fat". What they don't say clearly enough is that all meat contains predominantly saturated fat, even the *perceived* leaner meats such as chicken, turkey, and pork. What they don't say clearly enough is that those harmful saturated fats, in combination with animal casein* is about the equivalent of pointing a gun at your head.

Of course they don't say that, if they did the entire cattle industry in the US would cease to exist. Newsflash: it's coming. The upper echelon in our government may not be willing to admit this blatant reality in the next 5 years, it may not even be in the next 10 years, but it's coming...and if you want to live to see it, keep reading.

21

The information America is given about what is healthy and what is not is so convoluted and confusing that we look to the experts to help us. Who are the experts? Certainly not the marketing department of the largest food manufacturers in the country.

Do you think they care more about how their product affects your health or about how to get you to buy it so they can keep their job? There are people who report on certain scientific studies (the results of which are not actually proven more useful, but instead proven *less harmful*). Are those the people you're listening to?

What about the pharmaceutical studies where the drugs are compared against each other, and not against alternative treatments? This is supposed to be the guiding force? You certainly can't have unbiased, reliable information if a research study is conducted by people who are compensated by the very industry that they are performing research on! Remember the Enron scandal? In plain vanilla terms, the same institutions that educate our doctors of medicine are essentially held by the stature of the pharmaceutical giants that produce the drugs that supposedly cure us. How about that for transparency? Gosh there goes my cynicism coming out again. This is just another way in which confusion is perpetuated; how many more pharmaceutical advertisements do we have to watch on television suggesting we consult our doctor to see if a particular drug is right for us? I believe the term these days is "a pill for every ill".

---

*Animal casein is dietary protein found in all animal products, including meat, dairy milk, and eggs. It has been proven that adjustment of this protein intake is capable of influencing the ability of a chemical carcinogen to promote cancer.[2]

The discussion on corruption within these industries is quite political at the very highest levels, and certainly not what is most important in this book; the scandals are merely a devastating account of how the self-interest of America's largest industries influence and compromise government regulation on nutrition policy. This becomes important to understand, because as I will illustrate in the chapters to come, following the standard advice of medical practitioners requires not only reading between the lines, but perhaps more importantly, knowing what kinds of questions to ask. This shouldn't have to be the case. Transparency is required in financial and insurance dealings, in legal dealings, and in politics; it should be required in the food and medical industry too. America's chronic illness is keeping every health practitioner and pharmaceutical company in business.

Remember, education is about seeking all the information from every angle, evaluating these different perspectives, and then deciding how you will feed your family.

Part II
How to get past
the Health Crisis in America

CHAPTER 3:
A FOUNDATION TO MOVE FORWARD

There are a growing number of Americans, like yourself, who do care about what they eat and what they feed their children. We do care about putting apples and vegetables in our grocery carts instead of kool-aid and pop tarts, but it's imperative that we truly understand how certain foods differ so significantly from others, and why it matters so much. Reading the label will only give you the necessary information if you know *precisely how to read the label*. If you think label reading is slightly confusing, rest assured, after reading this chapter you'll feel much better.

Did you know that the United States government doesn't actually regulate what food manufacturers write on the front of their product packaging? In order to explain this, I want to start out by showing you the misleading marketing habits of the largest food manufacturers in our country...in enough detail that you will be able to make sense out of your grocery store and understand exactly what is suitable for your family to consume and what is not.

While the industrialized food chain is concerned with labeling and packaging, trying not to mislead the public about partially hydrogenated vegetable oil, what Americans need to realize is that the partially hydrogenated vegetable oil is one of the most likely causes of these diseases yet. So while the unknowing consumer focuses on looking at the amount of calories or carbohydrates in a particular product, we miss out on what the most important part of the label really is. What is the most important part of the label?

For starters, you should never believe what you read on the front of any product packaging.

Now that you know the regulations surrounding exactly what food manufacturers are allowed to place on the front of the package is not very heavily regulated, when you see something that reads "heart healthy" or "all natural" or "no artificial flavors" you now know why those words are extremely misleading, because those words are *not adequately regulated.*

WORDS LIKE THESE

ARE NOT ADEQUATELY REGULATED:

- Heart Healthy
- All Natural
- No Artificial Flavors
- No Artifical Colors

Here is another interesting fact that the food industry doesn't want you to know about: companies must pay a fee to use the American Heart Association's checkmark (logo) on their packaging. This is why the logo may appear on some products but not other products, even when both products meet the guidelines. Furthermore, the American Heart Association Checkmark specifically indicates that a particular food meets the criteria for saturated fat and cholesterol, so the food might contain a cup of high fructose corn syrup or refined sugar and still display the logo. So, the front of the package makes it seem healthful, but in actuality, it is not healthful at all. Isn't it interestingly deceptive when a product such as yogurt or ice cream claims that it is "gluten free"? Really? I didn't realize whole wheat, rye or barley was supposed to be an ingredient in dairy products in the first place. Of course it's gluten free.

28

The nutrition fact label and the ingredient list are what you need to look at. However, most of us look at the number of grams of fat or carbohydrates and assume we can make an educated decision about whether the product is healthy or not. Unfortunately, just looking at those two numbers is not enough. Oh, but you eat things in moderation? So did I. The reality is, moderation alone is not going to move you and your family toward better health. The running joke is, *Moderation* is a town we bypassed years ago; today, we all live in the town of *Excess.*

We all know we're supposed to cut back on refined flours, sugary drinks, and processed foods, but I have yet to hear someone make a claim as bold as "sugar causes cancer" or "margarine causes heart disease." Instead, people still believe margarine is the healthy alternative to butter simply because the packaging says "99% less fat". Advertisements like those, with little logos prominently displayed on the front of a package, make regular people believe that the spread is the healthier alternative when in actuality, that claim is 100% untrue. In fact, that 99% fat free spread is really 99% disease causing saturated fat. Maybe it's because our grocery store has a sign near the freshly baked bread that says "made with olive oil" so we perceive that to be better than the alternative. Or perhaps we see television commercials encouraging our children to eat a healthy breakfast, yet the visual is a child drizzling sugar on a breakfast toaster product. In reality, that product has had every last nutrient stripped out of it, and so have most of the cereals in your grocer's cereal aisle.

Most of the ingredients in the products we buy are unpronounceable. While our government has launched an all-out focus to make sure product packaging includes information about the ingredients, society has missed the most important part.

When we hear the term "processed" foods, we automatically think spam, hot dogs, or the cheese that you buy in individually wrapped cellophane paper. In reality, almost anything that comes in a package is a processed food item. This is the guiding force: if it comes in a package, then it is not good for you.

Foods that we eat every day, foods that we believe are healthier choices like whole wheat crackers, cereal, even yogurt, all of these are processed foods. While people are led to believe that certain processed food choices are better than others, the fact still remains that processed is processed. In simple terms, when a potato chip comes in a package, whether it is fried or baked doesn't really make much of a difference, there is no nutritional value in either of them when the second ingredient is oil. Have you ever read an ingredient label and wondered if you could break down all those separate ingredients at home to replicate that exact same potato chip? The idea of breaking down ingredients in order to isolate each separate item one by one is known as the concept of scientific reductionism. In other words, with foods that contain more than one ingredient (anything that is *not* a whole food) scientists can literally "reduce" the foodlike item to each additive, one by one. In fact, this is exactly how the vitamin industry came about. More on vitamins later.

Let's take a look at why the potato sits stagnant, quiet, and lonely in the produce aisle while the 100% whole wheat cracker garners the attention in the mid-section of the grocery store. Some popular trends in American society point the public in the general direction of choosing whole grain carbohydrates over refined carbohydrates. While this is true, what fly's in one ear and out the other, is the significant difference between plant based "complex" carbohydrates and simple "sugar" carbohydrates which is mostly what you find in the processed crackers and breads.

A complex carbohydrate is a macronutrient that your body needs for sustained energy while a simple carb is a sugar that causes an immediate spike in blood sugar and then almost just as immediately dissipates.

The perception is that a food like a whole wheat cracker, a granola bar or a protein bar, made with a whole grain such as oats, is a complex carbohydrate. This is only partially true. While one small processed ingredient may in fact be a whole grain, what you need to know is that the other 98% of the ingredients are simple sugars or additives that do more harm to your body than good. Have you ever noticed that you may eat a granola bar or a protein bar and then you are hungry an hour later? The reason is because the amount of sugar and artificial chemicals in the bar trick your blood sugar. This is precisely what the food industry wants to happen...buy that package of protein bars, and then become hungry an hour later so you can buy more of another packaged product. Remember, the simple reality is, there are minimal guidelines when it comes to food packaging. The largest food manufacturers no doubt have deep marketing budgets, and their advertising agencies have some creative folks who work there. They think you're going to equate the phrase "low-fat" with "healthy" and forget about all the unrefined sugar the product contains.

As a general rule of thumb, if a product has an actual label and the label contains more than 4 ingredients, it is a processed food item that is most likely not good for you.

Even if the label says "Made from 100% whole wheat" it is not a whole food because:

1. It comes in packaging.
2. It has more than one ingredient.
3. It does not grow naturally from the ground or on a tree.
4. Whole wheat is claim that is very different from "whole grain"

The best way to gain a better understanding about how to read ingredient labels is to follow some guidelines which I first heard about from someone who used to work for one of the largest food industry giants in our country. Jeff Novick currently serves as Vice President of Health Promotion for Executive Health Exams International and lectures at the McDougall Program in Santa Rosa, CA as well as the Engine 2 Immersion programs. Here is what you need to know about reading ingredient labels:

JEFF NOVICK'S RULES FOR
READING INGREDIENT LABELS

1. Do not believe what you see on the product packaging.

2. Read only the nutrition facts and the ingredient list.

3. The ingredient list contains the product's ingredients from most to least, so the ingredient listed first is the largest amount. In other words, if sugar, high fructose corn syrup, or brown-rice syrup is listed as the second ingredient, guess what that product is mostly made up of?

4. Fat: Don't try to break down the different types of fat in a product, they are listed in a deceptive way

and it does not help you make an informed decision about whether the product is healthy or not.

5.   Carbs should be only whole grain. Don't mis-read a label that says "100% Whole Wheat". Look at the list of ingredients. If the first ingredient is "White Wheat Flour" then there is nothing "whole" about it....it's not the carbohydrate intake that is the problem, it's the white flour, white sugar, white rice, and white pasta which have been refined to the point where all of the nutrients are stripped out of them and there is nothing left but "bad" carbs. The ingredient label must contain the words: whole, rolled, stone-ground, or cracked when referring to grains.

6.   Sugars: Avoid all added sugars. That's a tough one. If you must add sugar, try Maple Syrup or Agave in very small amounts. While the body needs simple sugars, they should only be gained from fresh fruits. Don't be fooled by thinking your body needs an "energy bar" as a simple sugar snack right before a workout...that is simply not true. The reality is, you should eat fresh fruit instead! Avoid any food with a label that has a sugar listed in one of the first 3 ingredients (and note that sugar, high fructose corn syrup and brown-rice syrup are all different ways of saying sugar).

Salt and fat require a little more of an explanation. So many of us try to avoid "adding" salt to a fresh vegetable. Maybe it's because our doctor told us we need to cut back on salt.

The Institute of Medicine (a branch of the National Academy of Sciences) acknowledges that 90% of Americans consume a harmful level of sodium every day. The human body needs only 2500 mg of sodium per day, according to the USDA Center for nutrition policy.

Let me put that into perspective: if all you ate were fresh fruits and vegetables, then you would be getting 5000 mg of sodium per day. But the kicker is, have you noticed how much sodium is contained in just one serving of a packaged food product?

I don't know why most people worry about a mere sprinkle of salt on a fresh tomato and basil salad when one handful of "whole grain" crackers or a few bites of a packaged product that poses as a healthy lunch like contains 10 times that amount! The next time you read an ingredient label, check out how much sodium *just one serving* contains. If you ate an entire can of tomato soup, for example, check the label to see how many servings of soup are in one can. Oh, 2.5. How many mg of sodium in one serving? 480. Oh, but, well, that was a small can of soup, so you ate the whole can which wasn't just one serving it was 2.5. Did you just consume 200 mg of sodium? Yes, you did, in one meal. And you're still hungry. Oh, so you don't actually eat cans of soup, but sometimes you cook with soup because you saw someone on television demonstrate how easy it is to make a quick meal. Cream of Mushroom Soup? Check out that can of soup. 870 mg of sodium per serving. 1 can contains 2.5 servings. 870 x 2.5 = 2,175 mg of sodium. Yikes. That is nearly enough for one entire day in just one can of soup!

This is just so fascinating that I have to examine one other packaged product that poses as being healthy to the average American. Let's look at tuna fish. A package that is 6.4 oz of Albacore White Tuna with a label on the front that says "In Water" as well as a little heart logo on the front that says "Natural Source of Omega-3". This doesn't seem deceptive at first glance until you turn it over and look at the Nutrition

Facts. Serving size is 2 oz, so there are 3 servings in this "package."

Now I'm looking at the actual ingredients: white tuna, water, vegetable broth, salt, pyrophosphate (stabilizer to increase shelf life, in other words a preservative). So at first glance, that looks like it isn't so bad with just a few ingredients. But look at the sodium, 240 mg per serving. Suppose you used the whole package (a very small, 6 oz package) and made tuna salad out of it for a sandwich adding something like chopped celery and a splash of low-fat mayonnaise thinking it's a healthy lunch; you first have to realize that is 240 x 3 = 720 mg of sodium in just one tuna sandwich. Then, to boot, tuna is an animal product that contains casein. Who is it again that is telling us to eat fish? Yea. One more thing, on the back, there is a little logo from the American Heart Association that indicates the product meets American Heart Association food criteria for saturated fat and cholesterol for people over the age of 2. Remember what the food industry doesn't want you to know...that logo is available to be purchased, that's right, for a price. Any product can display it proudly, as long as they pay for it. Tricky.

Getting back to label reading and what is actually stated on ingredient labels. Calories and Fat, but it is not clearly stated as a percentage, which is the math you need to do in order to actually figure it out. This is how those catchy bags of corn chips or yogurt can proclaim that they are 98% Fat Free on the label. What you need to do is long division. You need to know the amount of total fat in one serving as a percentage of total calories, and that is not directly provided to you as a number on the nutrition fact label. In reality, the label is *painstakingly* misleading.

There are 3 different units of measurement on that nutrition label: calories, grams, and percentages. The label gives you the total number of calories per serving and the total number of fat as grams, but the confusing part is that the total amount of fat is based on a percentage of total calories, not on grams, so you have to do the math.

I know what you're thinking: "I still don't get it." Yeah. That is exactly what the food companies want…for you to *not* get it.

This is how to calculate the real percentage of fat on an ingredient label:

1. Locate the number of calories per serving.
2. Locate the calories from fat, per serving.
3. Locate the number of grams of fat. A trick to make the math easy is to multiply the grams of fat by 10 because it is a measurement of weight. This now gives you the number of calories in each serving that comes from fat.
4. Divide the fat calories by the total calories to get the percentage of fat per serving.

Here is an example using a serving of crackers.

1. The number of calories per serving is 140.
2. The number of calories from fat is 45.
3. The number of grams of total fat per serving is 5, so lets multiply by 10 so we get 50, which is our number of calories in each serving that comes from fat.
4. If you divide 50 by 140, you get 35.7%. That is 35.7% fat per serving. A far cry from thinking you are getting a cracker that is 98% fat free isn't it?

The best way to accurately explain how ingredient labels mislead us by using terms like "98% Fat Free" is in this excerpt from a lecture by Jeff Novick:

> ...So you go to the grocery store and you say: "I can figure this out," and you pick up a product and you look at the nutrition facts label, figuring the government is making this easy for you. You say, "Okay, let's see what we have here." First thing you see is calories from fat, 20. Maybe you know what to do with that, maybe you don't. Then you see total fat, 2 g. Maybe you know what a "g" is or maybe you don't, but you're glad there are only two of them. Then over here it says 3% of a daily value. So they're listing fat three different ways by three different systems in one section. Is that helpful or confusing? Do you think that's done by accident?...

I was fortunate enough to hear Jeff Novick's lecture in person, in upstate New York during the summer of 2012. He used to work for Kraft Foods, one of the largest, industrialized food manufacturers, so he really has first hand knowledge about ingredient labels and has a humorous and candid way of getting a crowd to really understand how to interpret the label. He goes on to speak about the '80s, and how food manufacturers could actually get away with cheating on the nutrition label. This is how it works: if you buy a box of crackers and a serving contains 100 calories, the serving is 50% fat. But check this out, if you add some sugar (or honey or brown rice syrup) then the calories go up but it appears to reduce the amount of fat per serving. Now the food manufacturer can put a label on the front of the box that says "50% less fat per serving". So the average consumer thinks, hmm, that sounds good, oh, and since it's 50% less fat per serving, then maybe I should have a few more servings, heck, I'll just eat the whole box.

The other striking example to really drive the point home is oil. A tablespoon of oil is 120 calories, 120 calories, all of which are from fat. So if that oil was in a tiny container, the product would be 100% fat. But since everybody wants low-fat products and you've got a product that's either high fat or all fat, now you're stuck. According to Jeff, food manufacturers either have to make a better product or cheat. Guess what they did? They added water. Water does not have any calories or any fat. But does water have weight? Yes! It adds 750 grams. So the total on your ingredient label for olive oil is now 764 grams. So if you take the weight of the fat and divide by the weight of the serving, you can sell this 100% fat product as 98% fat free by weight. Hmm. My olive oil says that 1 tablespoon contains 21% of my daily recommended value of fat. Oh, but it's carb free. Onward with the cynicism: maybe you should consider just eating the olive instead.

Isn't it easier to just eat a whole food than worry about all the salt, sugar, and fat in the packaged product? Luckily these days we're all walking around the grocery store with a smartphone that has a calculator, but who has the time to calculate every nutrition label? Well, there are some books out there that can help you with understanding the lesser of two evils if you are still going to consume packaged products. I like a little manual called "*Eat This Not That*" by David Zinczenko and Matt Goulding. But, buyer beware. While these food swaps may help you choose the lesser of two evils when it comes to processed foods, the substitutions alone **will not** lead you down the path of disease prevention. Which warrants a discussion about...

CHAPTER 4: WHOLE FOODS

What exactly is a "whole food"? Part of my gripe with many of the books out there is that the author doesn't take the time to thoroughly explain, in simple terms, some of the most simplistic yet important concepts. What ends up happening is that people either get annoyed with reading something that takes a lot of effort to process (like standard deviation) or they fall asleep reading a book that is even more boring than a youth baseball game.

A whole food is a food that has one ingredient. If it looks like a carrot and tastes like a carrot, it is a carrot. A carrot is a whole food. A banana is a whole food. A potato is a whole food. All fruits and vegetables, in their "whole" form are whole foods. I digress for a moment; the tiny processed carrots that are pealed and shaped like a rounded nugget and taste like the plastic bag they came in are not the same as what I call "the bugs bunny" carrot that actually has a skin on it. As my 4-year old son puts it: "that carrot has hair on it." That "hair" is actually the most nutritious part of the carrot; so scub those carrots with a little soap and water, and a vegetable brush, and then eat it with the skin on it! We love the purple carrots. Do a taste test. I'm serious. You know you did the taste test of Coke vs Pepsi. It's time to try it on your vegetables.

For now, though, we need to differentiate between what is a whole food and what is not a whole food so you understand that very important distinction moving forward. A wheat berry is a whole food, but a "whole wheat cracker" you guessed it, is *not* a whole food. What is a wheat berry? It is a whole grain in its "whole" form.

Most Common Whole Grains

- Amaranth
- Barley (Gluten)
- Buckwheat/Whole Wheat (Gluten)
- Millet
- Oats
- Rice
- Rye (Gluten)
- Spelt
- Quinoa

The concept of exactly what a "whole food" is seems pretty simple, but I like to break it down because sometimes we still get sucked in to the commercials and advertisements which we already established are misleading. Hence the questions about whether a whole wheat cracker is actually good for you. In a cracker, most, if not all of the whole grain has been stripped away during the refining process.

This is another problem of late that perpetuates confusion, and it has to do with the grocery store's "organic" aisle. It is important to differentiate between organic and non-organic, but it is also important to remember, that packaged products are still packaged products. Just because a packaged product claims to be organic does not make it a health food. Keep in mind that counting calories methods are used by people who are opposed to eating the right foods, and this is quite possibly why so many people are misinformed. Diet systems like Nutrisystem and Jenny Craig help you overcome your weight problems in a motivational way with a "coach". It turns out that plans such as these are actually a very lucrative marketing business where the diet "system" promotes their own food, vitamin supplements, or people who are your personal cheerleaders… all with the intention of getting your money. Learning to eat the proper foods will help you bypass all the expensive brands that sell glamour instead of real food.

Let's go back to the basics: it's about understanding the impact of what you put into your body, not paying a monthly fee for pre-packaged TV dinners to be delivered to your door or for vitamin supplements that claim to have the magic ingredient. I have heard some diabetics use this common phrase "I can eat that as long as I take my insulin shot." That, in my mind, is like saying "This dessert might strip 20 years off my life, but I don't care, I feel good at the moment, it only has 2 points, and it tastes good for right now." And then there are the people who advocate "everything in moderation." I am familiar with this term…I used to subscribe to it. The absolute truth is, if you eat the right types of food, you can eat as much as you want and still maintain optimal health and optimal weight. Some people might call this belief over the top. I call cutting off a woman's breast over the top.

IF YOU EAT THE RIGHT TYPES OF FOOD, YOU CAN EAT AS MUCH AS YOU WANT AND STILL MAINTAIN OPTIMAL HEALTH AND OPTIMAL WEIGHT.

How do you go about determining what the right foods are?

Fats have 9 calories per gram while carbohydrates and protein have only 4 calories per gram. In essence, eating fresh, healthy greens actually reduces the calories you consume even though you might eat more. This is a concept called *nutrient density*. The most nutrient dense foods are plant-based. So just put weight loss goals to the side for a moment; if your ultimate goal is to feel better, live longer, look younger, lower cholesterol, prevent arthritis, stroke, surgery, kidney stones, cancer, and Alzheimer's disease, then ramp up your consumption of these nutrient dense foods and stop your consumption of EDNPF.[33] What the heck is EDNPF? Oh, it's the scientific name for junk food. You know…Energy Dense Nutrient Poor Foods, like the olive oil in your salad dressing, or the brown-rice syrup in your protein bar. But I thought olive oil was healthy? I know, so did I. I'm getting there.

First and foremost, the path to feeling better is not only about what you put in your mouth, it is about a lifestyle. In the twenty-first century, our lifestyle revolves around technology, and many urban and suburban home styles revolve around the kitchen. It's evident in the "open-layout" style of homes where people want their kitchen open to their family room so everyone can socialize, do homework, eat, and mingle together. We've already set the stage for family gathering in the kitchen, the hub of the home. Now it's just about educating ourselves on the right ingredients to make sure what we feed our family is the highest quality option.

Pasta, The Veg vs the Vegan

Unless you eat a whole food that is actually a real source of a complex carbohydrate such as a fruit or vegetable, then you are truly missing out on the whole point of the carbohydrate discussion. Being a runner, I often hear people talk about "carb loading" before a race. This is the perfect example surrounding those of us who "think" we're eating healthy but really need to understand and evaluate whether we are truly getting the intended benefit.

The idea behind carb-loading for the endurance athlete stems from the need for the body to use stored sugars called glycogen after the simple sugars in the body are used up in order to sustain performance. Remember though, good simple sugars are not found in "energy" bars, they are found in fresh fruit. Probably one of the most important parts about this glycogen conversion is that it doesn't apply unless you are performing more than 90 minutes. In other words, for the average 5k or even 10k race, it's highly unlikely that a person would need to "carb-load". In fact, carb-loading for a shorter distance is likely to promote weight gain, especially if you are using refined carbs such as bread, pasta, rice, cereal, and pancakes. While whole grains are part of the equation for "complex" or "good" carbs, they are not the full equation and need to be supported with other complex carbohydrate sources such as starchy vegetables.

Let's examine pasta for a moment. This is a tough one to swallow for me...someone who comes from a traditional Italian background. I know what you're thinking, Murray sounds Irish, not Italian. Murray is my married name; I am of Italian descent, and likewise grew up in a Mediterranean food inspired kitchen.

We perceive that we're eating something healthy by selecting whole wheat pasta as compared to semolina pasta, yet, the benefit we are looking for, the complex carbohydrate contained in the "whole wheat" portion of the pasta is really rather *insignificant* as compared to a potato for example, that we overlook the simplicity of the potato and forget about the other vitamins and minerals which naturally occur in a product of nature rather than a product of human synthetic production like pasta. In simple terms: even the whole wheat pasta is still a *processed* food. The nutrients in whole foods work together as if they are a symphony, they get absorbed and then become integrated in the body (we call this metabolism). This harmony of digestion is what *real nutrition* is really all about. Yes, whole grain sprouted pasta is better than semolina, but it's not as good as the potato.

Let's look a little closer at digestion. The process of the digestion of what we eat is such an incredibly complex phemonenena, that even in the twenty-first century the most highly educated scientists and medical doctors still have not even broken the tip of the iceberg when it comes to understanding how the human body processes nutrients. This is precisely why, to use a metaphor again, the whole [food] is *not the same* as the sum of its parts. In other words, while we have certainly been able to pinpoint that eating a handful of fresh berries provides a high concentrated source of vitamin C, we also know that an incredible amount of things happen when we eat the whole berry, and it is far from the same as taking a vitamin C tablet as a supplement. In other words, the vitamin industry as a whole is merely another extension of our processed food industry. Huh? Yes, it's true. Science has discovered how to isolate one single nutrient and literally "process" it into a capsule.

The part that tends to get overlooked by most of us when it comes to understanding the relationship between taking a vitamin versus eating a whole food is that our bodies produce an incredible acknowledgement of the whole food, so much more than any one vitamin capsule could ever replicate. Thousands of reactions and interactions occur in the cells of the human body in response to eating a whole food. Chemical reactions within human beings produce and unlock incredible amounts of vitamins, minerals, essential amino acids and components which we as a society have only just begun to understand, and could never replicate in one capsule. Taking one vitamin in isolation (a vitamin C supplement for example) can in no way, shape, or form, compare to eating a whole food. Have you ever read something like "you'd have to eat 45 servings of blueberries to get the vitamin C in one pill of X." That statement is a fabulous example of sensationalism; a journalist who has read one research study and fabricated a myth so far out of context that it just perpetuates public confusion...just to be the first to "break the story". In actuality, a blueberry contains some of the highest naturally occurring antioxidants of any food, as well as a host of other nutrients that are unlocked within the human body only after eating the whole blueberry; this simply cannot be replicated with one isolated nutrient in a processed, capsule form.

The premise behind the vitamin industry is of course intended to be a good way for human beings to supplement important vitamins and minerals that we may otherwise be deficient in if we are not getting enough in our diets. So we again come back to the fact that eating processed foods is the sole reason why our bodies are so deficient in these important vitamins and minerals in the first place. Try looking at it from another angle: when the human body is deficient in one vitamin or mineral, it is usually deficient is *all* vitamins and minerals. The same works in counterbalance: when the human body contains a sufficient amount of whatever vitamin or mineral you believe you're deficient in, all the other deficiencies soon are no longer deficiencies.

Think about this for a moment: we perceive that people who take vitamins have better health. Isn't it interesting, though, that the particular group of Americans, the middle and upper-middle class who can afford to buy the vitamins, tends to be the same group that also cares about their health enough to regularly exercise and eat a healthful diet?

The biggest indoctrination of scientific reductionism in America yet is the way the food industry has actually managed to "fortify" (synthetically add) vitamins to something like artificial sweetener. But that is a discussion for another day. In a nutshell, what you need to know about artifical sweetener is that *all artificial sweetener is poison*. I don't care how "natural" the commercial looks (marketing 101), the simple point is: avoid every single artificial sweetener at all cost. A sprinkle of sugar in your coffee is not what is making you fat and sick; it is the 20 teaspoons of artificial sweetener in your whole grain, low carb, vitamin B fortified serving of 10 ranch flavored 100 calorie cracker chiplike product that is really causing you harm! Fabulous. To drive the point home one last time, let's look at the following series of charts which should help clarify why eating one whole food can simply not be replicated with a processed capsule (vitamin).

Nutrients in Blueberries (Raw, 1 Cup)

Protein	1.1g
Carbohydrate	21.45g
Fiber	3.6g
Sugars	14.74g
Calcium	9mg
Iron	0.41mg
Magnesium	9mg
Phosphorus	18mg
Potassium	114mg
Sodium	1mg
Zinc	0.24mg
Vitamin C	14.4mg
Thiamin	0.05mg
Riboflavin	0.06mg
Niacin	0.62mg
Vitamin B-6	0.07mg
Folate	9mcg_DFE
Vitamin A	4mcg_RAE
Vitamin E	0.84mg
Vitamin K	28.6µg

Source (for all 3 charts):
U.S. Department of Agriculture. "USDA Nutrient Database for Standard Reference." Washington, DC

Nutrients in One Medium Apple

Vitamin A - 98 IU
Vitamin B1 (thiamine) - 0.031 mg
Vitamin B2 (riboflavin) - 0.047 mg
Niacin - 0.166 mg
Folate - 5 mcg
Pantothenic Acid - 0.111 mg
Vitamin B6 - 0.075 mg
Vitamin C - 8.4 mg
Vitamin E - 0.33 mg
Vitamin K - 4 mcg
Calcium - 11 mg
Copper - 0.049 mg
Iron - .22 mg
Potassium - 195 mg
Phosphorus - 20 mg
Magnesium - 9 mg
Manganese - 0.064 mg
Zinc - .07 mg

NUTRIENTS IN ONE SERVING OF SPINACH

	Macronutrients	
Water		Fat (Many Kinds)
Calories		Carbohydrate
Protein (Many Kinds)		Fiber
	Minerals	
Calcium		Sodium
Iron		Zinc
Magnesium		Copper
Phosphorus		Manganese
Potassium		Selenium
	Vitamins	
C (Absorbic Acid)		B-6 (Pyridoxine)
B-1 (Thiamin)		Folate
B-2 (Riboflavin)		A (as Carotenoids)
B-3 (Niacin)		E (Tocopherois)
Pantothenic Acid		
	Fatty Acids	
14:0 (Myristic Acid)		18:1 (Oleic Acid)
16:0 (Palmitic Acid)		20:1 (Eicosenoic Acid)
18:0 (Stearic Acid)		18:2 (Linoleic Acid)
16:1 (Palmitoleic Acid)		18:3 (Linolenic Acid)
	Amino Acids	
Tryptophan		Valine
Threonine		Arginine
Isoleucine		Histidine
Leucine		Alanine
Lysine		Glutamic Acid
Methionine		Aspartic Acid
Cyustine		Glycine
Phenylalanine		Proline
Tyrosine		Serine
	Phytosterols (Many Kinds)	

From the time I was a child, my parents instilled very traditional family values about food. I learned from a very young age that eating food at home with the family was healthier than going out to eat, and it cost less too. This was not the norm when I was growing up. People attended parties with store bought cookies and cupcakes or a "mix" where they added eggs and oil because either it was faster and more convenient, or they simply did not know how to bake it themselves. All across America, this is still the norm in some places, and it keeps growing stronger because the largest industrialized food companies promote unidentifiable chemical concoctions like icing that changes to any color you want.

In spite of all this, I believe the fundamental value of food has finally come full circle again, with modern families gathering in the kitchen, cooking together with our children, teaching each other about the importance of proper nutrition, and sitting together at the dinner table to discuss the day's events.

It took several decades before society finally got a handle on the fact that convenience doesn't win out over that which is most important, the good health of the people we care about most. We went from the idealism of the 1950s to the convenience of the 1980s when drive ins became drive throughs. We went from growing fruits and vegetables in our gardens to buying in bulk at large box retailers because it was more convenient and "seemed" less expensive.

Now, with the rise of word organic, we are finally beginning to realize that we *can* control our health with some very simple changes to our lifestyle. We're beginning to realize that it's not only hotdogs and candy bars, but *all* processed convenience foods are in fact the very products that are causing us to be fatter and sicker than ever before.

"I learned it by watching you." Some of us remember that one-liner from a tobacco commercial in the late '80s but conceptually, it makes a lot of sense. If adults model the behavior, children will follow suit. If I eat grapes, blueberries and apples for breakfast, then my children will eat the same. If I eat a bag of chips, my children will eat the same. It's not easy...lesson number 1: If you don't buy it, they can't eat it! Contrary to popular belief, children will *not go hungry* if you offer fruit and they don't eat it. If they are hungry enough, they will eat the fruit. It takes a lot of patience and discipline on the part of the parent. Believe me, I am living it myself.

Aside from labeling concerns, currently the USDA does not do a good enough job of warning us about the refined sugars that you find in almost all crackers, pretzels, graham crackers and chips. The increase in sugar consumption alone can account for the obesity epidemic. While scientists have come a long way in understanding the mechanisms by which calories from refined carbohydrates — fructose especially — have a disproportionate effect on weight and insulin resistance, the move toward eliminating those from our diets will probably take several decades to trickle down. Translation: our children eat too much junk. Basically, anything that comes in a box and has more than 4 ingredients is considered processed food. I'm not talking about spam here (well, that too) but I am talking about all of the snacks...graham crackers, cheese crackers, pretzels, corn chips. If it contains some form of sugar, salt, and partially hydrogenated vegetable oil in the first few ingredients, it is clogging your children's arteries and setting them up for disease.

The refined carbohydrate theory is only part of this equation though. Much research also points to animal protein, casein, as a leading factor in cell division. Looking at our healthcare system and the obvious need for changes, doesn't it logically make sense that the corruption exists because some industries stand to make or lose a lot of money? What if everyone in the United States stopped eating foodlike items that comes in a box? Some say that could never happen; but if it did, wouldn't you want to be around to see it?

I doubt our grandparents could have ever envisioned a world in which every 15 year old had their own personal mobile smartphone and easily communicated with people on the other side of the world. Isn't it remarkable that some of our elderly citizens, people born in the 1920s, once lived life without a television in their house? Over the last century, these people have lived through a whirlwind of changes in the world. We can only speculate about what the next 100 years will bring, but in the meantime, I think we all share one common dream and that is to lead a healthy life... at least long enough to see our children have children of their own.

Isn't it interesting how with just a little guidance, you can see how easy it is to make some small, but very important changes that will benefit you and your family for years to come?

4:11 am
I have to share this information now, with everyone I know, before it's too late! That's it. I'm doing it. I'm writing the book. I need to do this for my own children, so they know where they came from.

I truly believe this is what my mother would have wanted.

Chapter 5:
Partially Hydrogenated What?

While the USDA encourages consumers to evaluate ingredient labels before we buy (isn't it lovely that "buyer beware" now refers to food at the grocery store and not just real estate), unless we have a degree in biochemistry, none of us regular people really know the difference between expeller pressed sunflower oil and partially hydrogenated safflower oil...you know...the items you might find listed as an ingredient in your GMO-Free, Certified Organic High Oleic Corn Tortilla Chips. Uh, what?

It's the ubitiquous phrase that deserves clarification, partially hydrogenated vegetable oil; in its most familiar term, margarine. While butter contains saturated fat, the difference is that the saturated fat found in butter is naturally occurring while the saturated fat found disguised in most of the processed foods we know and love (olive oil included) is even more dangerous. The key is to understand why the difference is so important, then you can make an informed decision.

Hydrogenation involves adding hydrogen gas into vegetable oil under high pressure. This process makes the oil semi-solid at room temperature rather than liquid. What happens during the process of hydrogenation is that harmful trans fats are created which destroy the essential fatty acids and antioxidants that were otherwise present in the whole food (ie: the olive itself). Hydrogenation also slows spoilage, which is why you can leave the butter out on the counter instead of in the refrigerator, and it's also why you see the oil become solid in the refrigerator if you've stored leftover food that contains the oil you may have used to sauté it. Converting unsaturated (good) fats into saturated (bad) fats, with the process of hydrogenation, and then consuming, it is about the equivalent of poisoning yourself to death. Partial hydrogenation, while sounding like the lesser evil of full hydrogenation, still results in an increase in saturated fats for the end product. The theory is that most partially hydrogenated oils become more damaging to your health at high temperatures (such as when you fry potatoes to make french fries) because the heat releases the trans-fatty acids.

The common belief is that using monounsaturated oil like olive oil is the healthier choice. Not exactly. Olive oil still contains its fair share of saturated fat. While a better choice is thought to be an unrefined, cold-pressed oil like flax oil, what is the best choice? Do not use oil at all. Why? When any of the aforementioned oils are refined under heat and pressure, it is the refining process that actually damages it's omega-3 fats, and instead produces eruct acid (as well as the trans fats). Just a tiny sprinkle of these oils can produce devastating effects. Consumption of these oils is the most direct cause of heart disease and many cancers. Vegetable oils contain polyunsaturated fats, in very high quantity, in fact, just a tablespoon contains more than the average person should consume in a day. Think about how much oil is contained in a serving of tortilla chips. Look at the label, some type of oil is likely the second ingredient. If you think coconut oil, safflower oil, sunflower oil, olive oil, or flax oil is any better than canola oil…you are mistaken. With the exception of cold pressed flax oil, each and every one of these refined oils oxidize and produce free radicals in your body. It is these free radicals in which cancerous cells can easily bind to and multiply rapidly, and it is also these oils which lead to the devastating vascular diseases.

It is important to understand that the oils I am referring to in this discussion are refined oils, and not the naturally occurring oils in a product of nature such as the avacado.

That doesn't mean go out and eat only avacados for breakfast, lunch, and dinner, because although the fats and oils contained in an avacado are good and necessary, they should be consumed only in moderation by otherwise healthy children and adults.

Back to the unhealthy oils. Thirty years ago, the poster child was margarine; it was introduced when the federal government passed regulations that as long as a food product was labeled, it would be suitable to manufacture and market because full disclosure about the ingredients would be provided to the public. At the time, people didn't realize how deadly hydrogenation really would become. There are many ways to eliminate oil from the foods you eat: consider steaming vegetables, sauteeing in vegetable broth instead of oil, and using just vinegar on your salad instead of oil.

Before I started really researching ingredients, I just looked at the fat and carb numbers and called it a day, not realizing how incredibly dangerous it was to use oil. But, as we have seen so far…those numbers alone are definitely not enough to make an educated decision on whether the food is safe to consume.

Lets look a little closer at the process of hydrogenation: "trans" fats, trans referring to a certain configuration of hydrogen atoms in the fat molecules, are the substance used in many other types of processed foods that pose as being healthy, including tortilla chips which are perceived to be the healthier option to potato chips. Why are these other processed foods still perceived to be healthier? *The Journal of the American Dietetic Association* published an article[8] that indicated substituting foods rich in saturated fat with foods rich in high-oleic-acid sunflower oil has favorable outcomes. Unfortunately, this is what the public hears, what they don't hear, is that *the favorable outcomes* are specifically meant for people who previously consumed the higher saturated fat foods and simply replaced those foods with the lower saturated fat foods. So, let me interpret that for you. For people who eat a bag of potato chips a day, if they substitute a bag of corn chips fried in sunflower or safflower oil instead of potato chips fried in canola oil they might live 10 days longer than they would have if they continued eating the potato chips fried in canola. Safflower and Sunflower oils have higher burning temperatures. Realize that the food industry has become really good at replacing certain ingredients to another ingredient that is equally as unpronounceable to the average person, but, equally as *dangerous* to your health.

Since hydrogenation happens with so many of the products we consume, it's difficult to get away from. So what do you do? Stop. It's that simple. It is easy to get confused by foods that pose as being healthful because the front of the package says 'baked,' or 'low-fat,' or 'gluten free'. Unfortunately, if the second ingredient on the list is an oil well, that speaks for itself. Unfortunately our culture doesn't make it easy to just stop consuming snack foods all together. What is the lesser of two evils? Choose brands like Wasa, Ryvita, or another brand that is made with 100% whole grain. Rip Esselstyn's Engine 2 product line, available at Whole Foods Markets is another good choice of products to consider. Choose these instead of products where the first ingredient listed on the label is enriched wheat flour and the second ingredient is an oil. Even better, slice a fresh vegetable thin, with a mandoline, and bake it yourself with spices in the oven to create a crunchy snack food.

It is so important to really understand what you are reading on the ingredient label; once you do, you can clearly see why so many mainstream diet techniques just don't work.

AMERICA'S MAINSTREAM BELIEFS

Now that we have a better understanding of the fundamental flaw of oil, I would like to introduce you to the most provocative topic yet, the one fundamental, life altering detail that you may not have even been aware of until this moment: dairy.

Here is a little know fact: on July 19, 2012, a petition by the Physicians Committee for Responsible Medicine was filed in Washington, DC asking the U.S. Department of Agriculture to issue a report to Congress recommending an amendment to the National School Lunch Act...the amendment would exclude dairy milk as a required component of school lunches. Now we're getting somewhere. All animal based products, including dairy milk, cheese, meat, eggs, (even organic) as well as all fish contain an animal protein called casein; it is widely believed in the scientific research community that casein is the most potent chemical carcinogen of our time...even more potent than DDT and asbestos.[2] What?

ANIMAL CASEIN IS THE MOST POTENT CHEMICAL CARCINOGEN OF OUR TIME.

It is widely perceived that a glass of milk is a healthy option. Not only does dairy milk contain the millions of puss cells of animal casein, it contains saturated fat. Did you know that one glass of 2% dairy milk contains as much saturated fat as 3 strips of bacon? It's true. This is precisely why it's so important to properly understand the ingredients contained in the products you think are healthy so you can make an informed decision about what to put in your cart and on your child's breakfast cereal. The better choice is either Almond Milk or Rice Milk, for adults and children over the age of 2.

Try that little ingredient label trick we learned in the last chapter with the cup of cow's milk you put in your breakfast cereal each morning. Did you think you were getting 2% fat by choosing the 2% milk? In actuality, one serving of 2% milk is really 37.5% fat. Oh, and in case you were wondering, a serving of 1% milk is actually 25% fat and a serving of whole milk is actually 51% fat.

Yogurt is another perfect example. The yogurt that is marketed to children is especially problematic because it is made up of so many chemicals (not to mention antibiotics and hormones in the cows that are not grass fed) that it's a wonder why anyone would actually allow their child to consume something so dangerous. Look at the ingredient label on a product marketed as children's yogurt. Can you pronounce anything on that list? Do you even know what soy lectin or locust bean gum is? Remember how the U.S. Government doesn't want you to know about the harmful casein contained in all dairy products? Well, the casein is contained even in that "organic" children's yogurt. Not only is your child going to be hungry an hour later (just as if he ate a protein bar) but now all his other bodily systems have to work twice as hard to eliminate all the excess casein, sodium and sugar, so the child feels fatigue (which all parents know translates into the child being cranky and uncooperative). Wait, why does the body have to work so hard to eliminate the casein? Because it's not natural. It's not meant for human beings to consume, it's meant for baby cow's to consume. Why are you still drinking something that is meant for baby cows?

Just like the mainstream belief about cow's milk seemingly being a good choice, when you think about it, it's easy to see how those mainstream beliefs extend even further. Ahh, the high protein diet. Gosh but if you don't eat meat, where do you get your protein? Ahh. The high protein, low-fat diet. It's not Atkins, its South beach. Oh, but weight watchers helps you portion properly. Really? Is that because it's a TV dinner or a point system? I can put food on a plate with separate divisions for each food and call it proper portioning too. The raw foods diet. The vegan diet. The blood-type diet. It is so important to recognize why these diets are all fad diets and cause a host of other problems and are ultimately the cause of most chronic disease. The raw food diet and vegan scratch the surface of proper eating only slightly better than the others, but there is something called a "junk" vegan or "junk" vegetarian who may not eat meat, but instead consumes an abundance of other not-so-great additives, sugars, refined flours, soy products, and oils. Hmm, soy.

Before I dive into answering the protein question (this will be explained more thoroughly in chapter 10), I'd like to brief you on the second most asked question about food choices from people who still eat meat, and that is soy. Soy is high in phytoestrogens (plant-based estrogens that mimic estrogen in the body) as well as goitrogens (compounds that inhibit the thyroid's ability to correctly use iodine). Soy also contains hem agglutinin, a clot-promoting substance that causes red blood cells to clump together making them unable to absorb and distribute oxygen in the body. High levels of other harmful acids in soy reduces assimilation of calcium, magnesium, copper, iron, and zinc, and have been proven to cause growth problems in children.

If that isn't enough, trypsin inhibitors in soy interfere with protein digestion and cause pancreatic disorders. Some people experience irritable bowel syndrome after consuming products that contain soy. Free glutamic acid, or MSG, a potent neurotoxin, is formed during soy food processing increasing the body's requirement for vitamin D. Lastly, the processing of soy protein results in the formation of highly carcinogenic nitrosamines. Consider this, 91% of all soy grown in the U.S. is genetically modified. In other words, if your food comes in a package that has a barcode, there is probably soy in it. I'm not even getting into the genetically modified discussion (because that could be an entire book in and of itself). Google GMO and you'll see why.

Okay then, what about Asian populations who have been eating soy for generations? According to Kaayla T. Daniel, author of *The Whole Soy Story*, the Chinese first started eating soybeans about 2,500 years ago, but only after they figured out how to ferment it.[21] The fermentation process neutralizes the toxins in the soybean. Tempeh, miso, natto, and soy sauce have traditionally been fermented (although most soy sauce that you find in your grocery store is not).

Soy has it's place in the world, just not typically in my refrigerator, which is why I mentioned Almond Milks and Rice Milks earlier and not Soy Milks. I do use tamari, which is basically unrefined soy sauce, in my vegetable stir-fry, but I have also tried adding some garlic powder to extra firm tofu, using my hands to crumble it to the consistency of ricotta cheese and using it as a layer in my vegan lasagna. It certainly has the look and texture of ricotta, but coming from an Italian, lets just say it's probably better to forgo the ricotta layer all together. Here is what I think you should do...take soy in stride. As you'll see in the chapters to come, it is not easy to simply replicate the "standard American" menu in a vegan version. Instead, you'll learn to focus on recipes that celebrate the delectable plant.

Its frustrating watching friends, loved ones, and people all around us suffer from cancers, chronic degenerative conditions, diabetes, vascular diseases, and many more ailments where doctors cannot control the diseases with traditional medical therapy. Most people trust that physicians know best, and then instead of following a healthful diet, they go back to drinking cow's milk or eating those crackers that contain harmful oils because they don't even realize that is what is actually what is making them sicker. Many people don't always take the time to seek out alternative or integrative practices, where doctors of medicine focus on preventative healthcare instead of simply prescribing a band aid. It's so important to be aware, at this very moment in the twenty-first century, that even the vast majority of medical schools do not focus on diet and nutrition as part of their curriculum. Unfortunately, it's true, and I have personally confirmed this with many medical practitioners.

Some physicians, however, have been inspired by what they have observed. With a long list of credentials and many distinguished years of practice, one of those physicians is Caldwell B. Esselstyn, Jr., M.D., a former internationally known surgeon, researcher and clinician at the Cleveland Clinic in Ohio (ranked in the top 4 of the nation's hospitals by *US News & World Report*). Dr. Esselstyn has proven that even advanced cardiovascular diseases can be controlled with proper nutrition.[20] I had the pleasure of meeting Dr. Esselstyn in person, and later had the opportunity to discuss with him, at length, the remarkable findings in his research. You can find out more about the groundbreaking results of his 20-year nutritional study (the longest study of its kind ever conducted) where Dr. Esselstyn explains, with irrefutable scientific evidence, how people can end the heart disease epidemic in our country forever simply by changing what they eat. You can imagine my enthusiasm after that phone call! The name of his book is: *Prevent and Reverse Heart Disease*, by Caldwell B. Esselstyn, Jr. M.D. (2007).

It comes down to choice. We all have the choice to buy foods with multiple ingredients we cannot pronounce, or, we have the choice to buy whole plant foods.

In order to understand how people such as Dr. Esselstyn, Dr. Dean Ornish, Dr. John A. McDougall, Dr. Matthew Lederman, and myriad other physicians and scientists arrived at the idea that proper nutrition plays such a significant role in disease prevention, it's important to, in the words of the late Steve Jobs, "connect the dots looking backward." While the study of nutrition can effectively date back to Hyppocrates, among the more modern steps taken to measure the effect of the American diet on disease was started with several well-known studies back in the 1980s. Over the last 30 years, there has been an increased focus within the scientific research community on the role of exercise and nutrition on health, athletic performance, and disease.

While most people clearly associate regular exercise with overall health and wellness, what seemed interesting to me was that even people I knew who were physically active and ate healthfully still seemed to have diagnoses of cancer or heart disease popping up ever more frequently. Sure, we know that smoking increases the risk of lung cancer or that consuming nothing but hamburgers and french fries increases the risk of heart disease. But what about someone who runs 50 miles per week and maintains a healthy diet? It is rather significant to cite this astounding research that only between 5 and 10% of cancer is hereditary.[9] Why haven't we heard that number before? Why is it, that people who have a history of breast cancer in their family are encouraged to get more frequent mammograms? In fact, some research proves that the actual process of getting the mammogram actually increases the risk of the cancer. So when does preventative care equalize?

In order to answer these burning questions, I set out to learn as much as I could about the topic so that I could educate my family, friends, and anyone who yearned to know more. What I found was truly astonishing, but the more that I thought about it, the more I realized how it made such perfect sense.

On the one hand, you have the physicians, the highest educated people in their field. They are hard-working and honorable people who strive to provide the highest quality of healthcare. On the other hand, you have basic economics, the free-market system, the American dream...the foundation upon which our country was built. The industrial food companies in the U.S. want to produce products with a shelf life. The only way to do that is to take the essential oils out of the grains. When something comes from nature, it's healthy, but when you refine and process it, suddenly it's a disease-promoting ingredient. Then the farmers want to produce crops that are bigger and better because the assumption is that those are the ones that sell, and the vicious cycle continues. Regular people just don't understand how significant the ramifications are of eating these foods. I still, to this day, witness people in the grocery store who select the largest, best looking strawberries, even if it's January. I think to myself, don't they know that tasteless fruit was grown with modified, synthetic methods and pesticides? The reality is, they don't know. Perhaps that is why they sprinkle sugar (or worse, some synthetic sugar substitute) on top of the berry, to make it taste "better".

By nature, we are not a pragmatic society. Our social world is made up of many systems, a stream of behaviors embedded in other systems. A collection of interrelated components involved in unique contexts. If we simply follow one of the golden rules of overall wellness and stop our busy lives for just one moment, we realize the overlap in personal and social systems that allows us to arrive at ethical and aesthetic judgments. Over the last 5 years, interest has grown exponentially in identifying strategies to reduce the risk of chronic diseases, everything from lifestyle and wellness intervention programs in the corporate arena to behavioral modification programs for children. By recognizing the connections between food and disease, we, as a society, can identify ways to better our health and quality of life. One way scientists can actually measure the impact of certain food on certain diseases is through clinical research on preventive and rehabilitative health.

This is exactly what was measured in the largest, most well-known study on human nutrition and the connection to disease, *The China Study.* Co-author, T. Colin Campbell, PhD, is a professor emeritus of nutritional sciences at Cornell University. I also had the distinct pleasure of meeting Dr. Campbell in person, and hearing him lecture about his lab expirements between the 1960s and the 1990s. A remarkably knowledgable gentleman and testament himself to the longevity of eating whole, plant-based foods. In his words, "...a biological symphony."

It turns out that in our society, sometimes the external laws of morality are actually what determine survival of the fittest, because society doesn't understand consequences. The consequences are that Americans have become so lazy that only those who take an active role in their own wellness will be the ones who thrive. Those who rely strictly on single-nutrient effects, whether it is modifying the fat content in the cheese by adding more water, and hoping to reduce cancer by mere wishful thinking alone, or whether by adding back a single synthetic vitamin during the refining process, we now know how easy it is for Americans to conform to information that has a fundamental flaw; the flaw is that the biggest industrial food companies have the biggest advertising budgets.

Labeling aside, the vast number of advertisements promoting unhealthy products as healthy options are the biggest culprits. Then comes our well-intentioned government. Instead of spending hundreds of millions of dollars on political campaigns that draw attention to the flaws of political candidates, we should be making sure our children are educated on proper nutrition. The school lunch program in the wealthiest country in the world is just plain embarrassing. The other governmental food programs...hospitals, educational programs for childbearing woman and their infants, and the industrial food labeling programs also contribute exponentially to the widespread epidemic of obesity in our country. These federal programs along with the education programs for doctors of medicine also have a fundamental flaw...think about it, who really controls the development and dissemination of diet and disease information within our society?

You guessed it: once again, the answer comes down to greed. Some of the most profitable industries, both public and private, in our nation are those that have the most control over what the American public sees, reads, hears, and follows. We live in a culture where people go to work because it's their job and not because it's their passion; they allow the desire for material wealth to outweigh the highest amount of riches that exists which is the health and happiness of those we love. The media reports to break a story rather than getting all their facts right, and some medical practitioners diagnose, order tests, and prescribe powerful pharmaceutical meds within 10 minutes of meeting you rather than carefully reviewing a lifetime of factors that potentially contribute to your condition.

It's no longer about differentiating between hydrogenated and partially hydrogenated oils. Or, for that matter, it's no longer about differentiating between red meat, poultry, or fish. We already know the only way to stop fueling disease is to eliminate the culprit. The answer to all this seems complex, but what it all really comes down to is educating one person, one family, one organization at a time on the benefits of eating only plant-based, whole foods.

These facts, which collectively I like to refer to as the "Silent Cure", have been proven over and over again for generations. Take your own "Plant Pledge" by following these basic guidelines:

The Plant Pledge

- Vegetables in their whole form provide the best source of protein and fiber for the human body to function optimally. Buy organic as much as possible.

- As a society, we consume an excess of harmful food additives as well as too much protein. Just stop. Stop all artificial sweeteners, and stop eating meat; there are no nutrients found in meat that you cannot otherwise get from vegetables.

- The powerful anti-oxidants in whole fruit are the single best way to eliminate toxins from the human body. Don't be the person who falls prey to the dietary "cleanse". You can adjust the alkaline balance in your body and naturally cleanse yourself by eating a serving of fruit each morning.

- Eliminate oil. This is the single hardest thing to do because oils in all their different forms are found in nearly every packaged product that exists. Stop eating processed foods that contain oil, or at least cut back significantly.

Got it? Next…the rules.

THE RULES OF THE
PLANT PLEDGE

What you CAN eat:

1. Whole foods that are a product of nature, not a product of industry. This includes fruits, vegetables, legumes, nuts, and whole grains.

2. Limit your beverages to water, coffee, tea, or fruit juices that you juice yourself only.

3. Snacks like dried fruit, seeds, and nuts

4. Natural sweeteners like honey, maple syrup in moderation

What you CANNOT eat:

1. No meat or dairy products, including milk, eggs, or cheese.

2. No refined grains such as white flour or enriched wheat flour.

3. No artificial sweeteners like Splenda, Stevia, or corn syrup.

4. Nothing out of a box, bag, bottle, or package with more than 5 ingredients listed on the label.

5. No "fast food" or deep "fried" food.

Check out the Recipes section in the back of this book, as well as my website for ideas! http://asilentcure.org/blog

Why not give this a try? Try it out for 10 days...you can do ANYTHING for 10 days! It costs you nothing but a little effort. I know you still have a lot of questions...so finish the book first! As we move along through the chapters, you'll find there are charts in the back of this book to help you make sense out of some of the substitutions that I talk about.

While it may take decades to come full circle on major issues such as U.S. Healthcare spending, agencies like the USDA long known to be subservient to the meat and dairy industry, or significant global issues such as sustainability of natural resources in the environment and world hunger, we have to begin somewhere, and that place is right here in your own community, in your own home. Invariably, the trickle-down effect is likely to last an entire generation before the politics involved in these high ranking programs actually enable them to institute change that will be beneficial for society as a whole rather than just a select few. Unless that is, Americans actually start using the free-market system that has worked so well for hundreds of years. You know what I'm talking about...good old supply and demand. If we demand organic produce, milk without hormones and antibiotics, and preventative healthcare rather than sitting back and waiting for someone to find the magic pill that will cure all disease, then maybe, just maybe we have a fighting chance.

Part III
The Rise of the Organic Generation

A Silent Cure in my Back Yard

70

CHAPTER 6:
FROM SOIL TO PESTICIDE

Fifty years ago, we didn't have to worry about whether food was grown organically or not; farms across the United States were intimately tied to their own communities where environmental stewardship was evident from the farm to the local markets where the goods were sold. Then, genetically modified crops, pesticides, and over-fishing our oceans won out over sustainability, and grocery stores from coast to coast began to stock everything from exotic produce to farm-raised fish. Exotic produce?

Hmm, even Brazil has stricter regulations than the United States. The term "GMO" stands for genetically modified organisms. In other words, in the United States, cattle farmers feed genetically modified corn to their cows because it is less expensive, and that is why the cattle are sick and need antibiotics and hormones to produce more of the milk and beef that the uninformed people of the United States consume every day. It's sad but true, the government spends our tax dollars to subsidize this type of industry, artificially lowering the cost of beef and chicken so people are willing to eat it, because it's an American industrial system. GMOs are a long and detailed discussion; of which I couldn't even begin to scratch the surface.

Ever since 1988, the European Union has prohibited the use of growth hormones in the raising of cattle while the United States Department of Agriculture has deemed growth hormones safe for cattle and thus, human consumption. Not only that, the Food and Agriculture Organization of the United Nations (UN-FAO) actually attributes 18% of worldwide greenhouse gases to the production and consumption of livestock.

Links have been established over and over again between the hormones used in cattle and premature development in girls, lower sperm count in men, and certain cancers. What is the common factor? Animal products, meat, dairy, and eggs. While grass fed cattle might offer you some hope, the truth is that *even organic meat carries the casein that is linked to tumor development.* When you see the term "low fat" and "heart healthy" and "all natural" on packaging, the claims seem believable, but as previously mentioned, that is exactly what the manufacturer is trying to do…they think you're dumb. In reality, these claims mean nothing because remember, the USDA *does not regulate* the use of those words.

Oh, and by the way, in case you missed it, in the spring of 2012, the USDA quarantined two dairy farms as a result of finding mad cow disease in their cows. They claim the cows and their offspring were "destroyed" before their products entered the animal or human food supply, but how do dairy cows get mad cow disease you ask? By eating the remains of other cows who had it. In order to prevent the spread of this disease, the USDA has outlawed this feeding practice, however, ahem, cow remains are rendered into protein pellets and fed to chickens. Then, the chicken feed is used to make industrial cow feed. Through this perverse food chain, infected cow remains can still find their way back into the diets of uninfected, factory-farmed dairy cows. If this cannibalistic animal feeding practice makes you sick just thinking about it, consider the fact that the quality of your dairy and meat products are directly related to the health of the animals producing them. That in and of itself is enough to make me buy organic.

If that isn't enough to turn your stomach, lets talk about fish for a moment. Oh you thought fish was better than meat? The term "farm raised" refers to a cramped pen full of sick, disease infected fish; does that make you want to eat those fish? The good news is, if you are a meat eater (including fish, which is still considered animal protein) then the magic number is 5%. If you can maintain 5% or less in your overall diet, then you can still eat a small serving of whatever meat or fish you choose now and then. By now and then...I'm talking about once a year, not once a week! Hmm. Ya. Moderation. Once you begin to feel the good effects of the plant-based foods, you will be less likely to resort back to animal foods anyway. The best method to make you a believer is to actually experience it for yourself. If you have high cholesterol and you thought you ate a healthy diet, consider trying out something different for just 10 days; take The Plant Pledge. Eliminate ALL meat, dairy, and eggs. I challenge you. Give it just 10 days and see if you feel better, see if you have more energy. But, and this is a big but...be honest about it. It's not easy to cut cheese out of the standard American diet! Believe me, I know, I've been there. And to be perfectly honest, you may catch me eating a serving of ice cream once or twice a year. I'll be under the boardwalk.

ORGANIC PLANT FOODS

VS.

REGULAR PLANT FOODS

Do you buy produce at your local grocery store or local farmer's market that looks picture perfect but tastes like the chemicals that were sprayed on it? Be careful of that produce, it contains little or no nutrients because it was genetically modified in an effort to lengthen the shelf life by 'turning off' the genes linked to the production of the enzymes that cause it to ripen. Oh, so that's why the fruit doesn't seem to taste like it's supposed to. Unfortunately, we even have to be aware of this when it comes to local farmer's markets, because these days, not all farmer's markets actually grow the food that they sell. Some of the stands are actually just trucking in their produce, the same way your local grocery store is. The best way to find out: ask! Ask if their produce is grown locally. Ask where it came from. Ask if it's grown organically, without the use of harmful chemicals.

The battle over a cancer causing pesticide often applied to strawberry fields is finally over. Arysta LifeScience, the maker of the highly toxic methyl iodide, pulled the agriculture pesticide from the market not long ago. I usually buy organic anyway, but if you currently buy those nice big strawberries at your market because they "look nicer," then this is good news for you! On a more serious note, if you have children, it is definitely worth paying the organic premium, especially on what they eat the most.

Organic foods taste the way nature intended, they are better for the environment (because they are produced without using synthetic pesticides and fertilizers) and they are the most nutritious foods to consume because organic fruits and vegetables are grown naturally, without antibiotics or growth stimulants. Essentially, the highest quality produce is grown both organically and locally, wherever it is that you live. When selecting produce, I cannot stress enough the importance of choosing fruits and vegetables that are in season in your area of the country, and buying from a local farmer. Better yet, grow it yourself. Nothing in the world tastes better than the strawberries from my neighbors patch in June or a tomato from my own garden in August. And people wonder why I picked 22 pounds of blueberries from my local orchard and put them in my freezer.

Interestingly, a recent Stanford University study[22] challenged the benefits of organic produce versus non-organic produce, but what was exposed instead was that one of the study's co-authors, who has a long history as an "anti-science" propagandist, also has ties to the tobacco industry, and further, the University has financial ties to Cargill, a powerful proponent of genetically engineered foods and an enemy of the GMO Labeling Proposition [37]. Scientific evidence actually demonstrates that the study was crafted under the influence of researchers pushing a corporate agenda, as it is well known that the co-author in question developed a "multivariate" statistical algorithm, which is essentially a way to lie with statistics (or to confuse people with junk science).[23] Hmm, well I guess that discounts that study now doesn't it?

Aside from the obvious growth hormones, organic food has little or no pesticide residues. This in and of itself is a big deal, especially if you merely give your produce a "rinse" before eating. I have become a bit obsessed about using soap to scrub my fruit and vegetables as soon as I get home from the market. I have also been known to give out a vegetable brush as a prize during my lectures on nutrition! I suggest using the vegetable brush often because a mere "rinse" is not going to wash off the pesticides. According to the Environmental Working Group (ewg.org) the most pesticide-laden fruits and vegetables are: apples, celery, strawberries, peaches, spinach, imported nectarines, imported grapes, sweet bell peppers, potatoes, blueberries, lettuce, and kale/collards. The "Clean 15" are: onion, sweet corn, pineapples, avacado, asparagus, sweet peas, mangoes, eggplant, cantaloupe, kiwi, cabbage, watermelon, sweet potatoes, grapefruit and mushrooms. (For easier reference later, I have included this information as a chart below and in the resources section in the back of the book.)

There is also a mountain of evidence that suggest produce grown in organic soil has higher levels of a variety of nutrients, including vitamin B12, and in fact, it is the state of the soil that really determines how well produce grows. Just look around, or "taste" around. The organic fruits and vegetables actually taste the way nature intended. The colors are bright and beautiful, and that is not by accident. The naturally occurring vitamins and minerals in fresh produce is not only what gives it the vibrant color, but also transfers from the plant to the human beings that consume it. These vitamins and minerals cannot be reproduced with scientific reductionism (meaning, by taking a vitamin supplement). The vitamin industry has capitalized on the very notion that scientific researchers have literally "reduced" complex food to an isolated equation, however, the whole food is simply not equal to the sum of it's parts; obviously we cannot take a vitamin and stop eating food.

Remember what happens when the whole food is digested…it is a miraculous biochemical process of nature that simply cannot be replicated in a vitamin.

THE CLEAN 15 ™

VS

MOST PESTICIDE LADEN

	Dirty Dozen		The Clean 15
1	Apples	1	Onions
2	Celery	2	Sweet Corn
3	Sweet bell peppers	3	Pineapples
4	Peaches	4	Avacado
5	Strawberries	5	Cabbage
6	Nectarines - imported	6	Sweet Peas
7	Grapes	7	Asparagus
8	Spinach	8	Mangoes
9	Lettuce	9	Eggplant
10	Cucumbers	10	Kiwi
11	Blueberries - domestic	11	Cantaloupe - domestic
12	Potatoes	12	Sweet Potatoes
		13	Grapefruit
		14	Watermelon
		15	Mushrooms

Plus: Green beans, Kale/Greens (many contain residues of special concern.)

Source: ewg.org

Headquartered in Washington, DC, the Environmental Working Group (EWG) is a team of scientists, engineers, policy experts, lawyers and computer programmers that uses government data, legal documents, scientific studies and their own laboratory tests to expose threats to public health and the environment, and to find solutions.

Community Supported Agriculture

You may have heard a lot about this relatively new acronym, CSA. What is it and why is it important to me? Community Supported Agriculture (CSA), is a national network of participating local farms across the United States which use organic or biodynamic farming methods, and strive to provide fresh, local, high-quality whole foods. The CSA actually had it's beginnings more than 20 years ago, with the Organic Foods Production Act of 1990. The term "high-quality" means food and/or livestock that is grown organically, without the use of pesticides or other chemicals such as miracle grow, growth hormones, or antibiotics. The largest CSA along the mid-Atlantic corridor is the Lancaster Farm Fresh Cooperative (LFFC). LFFC is a nonprofit organic farmers cooperative of 75 farmers (current as of the date of this publication) in Lancaster County Pennsylvania that provides USDA Certified Organic vegetables and fruits. The LFFC focuses on creating healthy high quality foods from highly maintained and enriched soils.

The Lancaster Farm Fresh Cooperative serves all of Eastern Pennsylvania, New York City, New Jersey and Delaware by connecting the farmer and customer, delivering the best local organic produce to well-known grocery store chains such as Whole Foods Markets, and also to retail establishments, co-ops, restaurants, and institutions in the Mid-Atlantic region. For residents local to this area of the country, there is even delivery service available. Some friends actually didn't believe that I had freshly harvested organic produce delivered to my door each week.

Freshly harvested produce through the CSAs across the country operate on a subscription program in which members commit to support their farmers for the entire growing season by paying for their share of the harvest in the winter and early spring. The farmers are able to purchase supplies in the winter and start their crops in early spring, they repay the shareholders in fresh, organic, seasonal produce. CSA enables you to keep your family healthy by consuming local sustainable products as you support both the environment and your local farmers who produce high quality crops that will be safe for future generations.

If you do not live in the Pennsylvania, New York, or New Jersey area, you can find a CSA near you through these two sources:

USDA National Agricultural Library
http://www.nal.usda.gov/afsic/pubs/csa/csaorgs.shtml

Local Harvest Database
http://www.localharvest.org/

There are a variety of reasons organic food costs more than conventional food. The demand for it far exceeds the supply, and organic farmers receive practically no subsidies from the government. When I asked one of my local farmers whether he would consider moving toward organic farming, his response was candid: "They [meaning the government] don't make it easy or profitable for us, so I don't foresee that happening."

European governments do subsidize the transition to organic, while our government does not. Why? While farming without chemicals is inherently more labor intensive, the CSA can help families like yours make better choices when it comes to fresh, locally grown produce.

CHAPTER 7:
MOVING CHILDREN FORWARD

We have heard this before...get your children involved in food preparation and build the foundation for proper nutrition early. Somehow, our priorities got flip flopped over the last generation. Somehow, people decided to put sugar on fruit to make it taste better; that is like putting a band-aid on a broken arm. Instead of getting to the root of the issue (why the fruit doesn't taste good is because it's laden with pesticides and void of nutrients) we disguise the taste with sugar.

In actuality, an organically grown strawberry, in season, tastes delicious without anything added to it. Just visit your local farmer's market in June for the best strawberries you have ever tasted.

In fact, many orchards allow consumers to pick their own produce. You can literally stop and smell the roses in your own life by taking a 5-year old to pick produce at your local orchard. Just sit back and watch how beautiful it is as this little person carefully and magically picks fruit herself and immediately eats it right off the tree. Right then and there, you are teaching that child an elaborate and secret code of ethics that is written nowhere, and understood only by a few. It is one of the great lessons of life, true gratitude for what nature intended. That is pure, unadulterated beauty.

We're being told that American children suffer earlier from the symptoms of diabetes, symptoms that experts suggest can be controlled by drugs. Children on drugs for the rest of their lives?

I'm not only talking about type 2 diabetes, I'm also talking about type 1 diabetes…similar diseases, yet vastly different in how each comes about. Type 2 diabetes used to be called "adult onset diabetes" until it started showing up earlier and earlier. Then the name was changed to type 2 diabetes. Type 2 is both preventable and curable with the lifestyle changes suggested in this book. At this point in time, though, scientists have not established a direct cause of Type 1 diabetes like they have with Type 2. Some studies suggest onset may be caused by the mother's diet during pregnancy, or the fact that infants were fed formula instead of the mother's breast milk,[31] while other current research suggests the disease is caused by a virus. Remember, in Type 1 diabetes, scientists are still not sure what specifically prompts the autoimmune response that destroys the body's ability to produce insulin. In some cases, only certain genetic predisposition is apparent, while in other cases, it is environmental factors that trigger Type 1 prevalence even more than previously thought; this of course is not explained by genetics.[32] Therefore, it should be concluded that it is more important than ever, both for Type 1 and Type 2 diabetics to pay close attention to the types of foods they eat, and the ingredients contained in those foods. Yet the question still remains: children on drugs for the rest of their lives?

Yes, it is true that doctors can control disease with prescriptions, and while these drugs can and do treat some of the symptoms, the problems lie in the fact that a pharmaceutical medication is treating, not curing the condition. It's time to get back to basics, why not do everything possible to help prevent the condition, especially if it can be accomplished by paying close attention to the types of foods you eat? It's no secret that diabetics need to pay close attention to the foods they eat, but think about this:

did you ever consider that the animal casein found not only in meat, but in dairy, cheese, milk, and cream could actually be making the condition worse?

The other part of the problem, as we mentioned earlier, is that Americans have a hard time getting their priorities in order. We spend more time, as a society, driving our children to sports practice because we're told that children need exercise. No doubt that is true, but if a child becomes so involved in the sport that you have to feed him a pre-packaged cereal bar (processed food with no nutritional value) because the family doesn't have time to eat a meal together, then is that contributing to the problem? What can we do about it? Well you've already begun the journey toward educating yourself on proper nutrition, so you can start off on the right foot by throwing away all the protein bars in your pantry and tossing out all the chicken nuggets in your freezer! At the end of this book, there is a chart with common substitutions to get you started on the path to better health.

I might be a little over the top, to the point where I sing "Take me out to the Ballgame" to my son but instead of saying "buy me some peanuts and cracker jacks" I sing "buy me some broccoli and carrot sticks". Yes, that's true too. This is part of the reason this book came about...because I felt like I needed to provide an in-depth explanation to my friends about how and why decisions about groceries significantly impact our own health and the health of our families. The magic of childhood is brilliant, and the most critical age of influence about food in children is from when they can eat solid foods, at about 9 months, until the age of 6. In those primary years, it's no secret that your child is most highly influenced by what you eat at home and by what they learn at school.

By the time my daughter was ready to begin kindergarten, she already knew that her lunch of a lettuce wrap, carrots, grapes and homemade, whole grain granola with plain water was healthier than processed chicken nuggets and french fries. Really, it's 2012 and nuggets are still on the menu. As of right now, this is what the USDA mandates on the public school system in our country. And the worst part is, many parents and school foodservice directors are not as well versed in plant-based nutrition as they should be. The ramifications of serving this type of food to school age students is horrific. The most disheartening part of the story is that people still think cheese and yogurt is a healthy snack. Obviously obesity in our country speaks for itself.

I was told that schools do not serve water because it is "nutritionally deficient". Wow. So milk laced with hormones and antibiotics or a flavored "juice drink" (read: sugar water) is better than plain water? Why should I expect the school to do anything different than make the best of their own operating budget, especially when every country except the United States of America bans the use of antibiotics and hormones in their cattle. Cheese has a story too, not only does it contain the harmful casein, hormones, and anti-biotics, but in many cases is subject to hydrogenation which changes the chemical composition even more. As a society we love cheese, and I'll be the first to tell you that cheese is one of the most difficult things to remove from your diet. You've got to find your way out of your misguided relationship with cheese; we all love cheese, but cheese simply does not love us back.

We strive to teach our children by example. We've all heard the term "do as I say, not as I do." At home, by example, this is where proper nutrition begins. Children are so impressionable, especially by the people they look up to most…the parents, grandparents, caregivers, and teachers; children eat what they are fed early in life. If those people are not on board, supporting one another through the process of educating children on what is appropriate to eat and what is not, then it just makes the job that much more difficult. We encourage communication about important life events such as changing jobs, getting married, buying a house, having a baby, and estate planning; when are people going to realize that you cannot plan for those events if you are not healthy. The health and wellness of a person, of a family, of a society starts right now, with each person reading this book. It's a commitment. One by one. Family by family.

One of my favorite sources for nutrition information over the years has been The Rodale Institute, a 501(c)(3) nonprofit dedicated to pioneering organic farming through research and community outreach. Check out their program for children "Grow It, Cook It, Eat It" www.rodaleinstitute.org. Also, to help round out your understanding on why current national dietary guidelines do not represent society's real beliefs about the best practices for nutrition, read *Solving America's Healthcare Crisis!* by Pam Popper, Ph.D., N.D.[24]

Because of the "guidance" that our children need more exercise, we have signed them up for so many extracurricular activities that the schedule for most families today actually prevents our children from being a child. Instead of focusing on doing things together as a family, we now focus too much on not being late for baseball practice 6 nights a week at the expense of eating a proper meal together as a family. We swapped out the apple for the energy bar, with the mistaken understanding that somehow, a processed, glorified candy bar could replace a whole food.

What happened as a result? Older children turn to the "energy drink" a chemical concoction of nastiness that is equivalent to drinking hairspray. We wonder why our small children are tired, cranky, and unwilling to behave properly. We wonder why our older children are disrespectful to one another and to authority. We no longer sit down together as a family for dinner because we're too busy making sure our older children get the "exercise" they need at the expense of the core value of the family unit.

I am certainly not suggesting that your child should not participate in extracurricular activities; I am simply saying that the key to a healthy lifestyle is 100% directly related to what you eat. Take a good, hard look at what you eat, at what you feed your children, and consider how nutrition really fits into your lifestyle. If you make it a priority, then your actions will guide your children to make it a priority. The road to lifelong health begins in childhood and balance begins in the home, so if you don't teach your children what is right from the beginning, then who will?

Life's greatest reward is always at the end of a journey of hard work and dedication. Eating clean is hard work because American culture has made it that way. The only way it will change is by each one of us making the choice to feed our family healthfully, and stand by that choice. It isn't about doing what is easy, it's about doing what is right. Stand up for carrots instead of cupcakes in your child's classroom. I did, and my community of parents stand by me. Sure, everyone has a birthday, but in a class of 30 students, that is a cupcake every Friday for the entire school year. If our schools are not reinforcing the appropriate behaviors we model at home, then who is? Somehow, our society continuously revolves around the easy way out. Sure, it's easy to buy a packaged product and then throw away the trash, but is it really worth it? Is that the behavior you want your children to follow?

CHAPTER 8:

GRATITUDE IS AN ART

Sometimes it takes something as powerful as life itself to force us to realize how fortunate we really are.

What is it with people who don't pay attention? Maybe it's a sign of contemporary culture, but in my mind, being understood means listening.

So I'm in the maternity ward, and the signs all over my hospital room say "Breastfeeding" so why does someone come in and give me a welcome package with 5 different samples of formula in it? How about some bags or bottles for my breast pump, or some lanolin cream for my sore nipples? What am I going to do with formula? I don't even have a bottle to put it in.

My daughter was born in the spring of 2007, I was in the hospital at the same time my mom was in another hospital about an hour away, awaiting her turn on the list of recipients for a bone marrow transplant. We donated my daughter's umbilical cord blood to the National Bone Marrow Foundation*. My mom underwent the transplant that summer, and because of her strength and determination, she finally came home. It was far from back to normal, but the miracle of my newborn baby brought an unexplainable amount of hope to our whole family.

---

* Current at the time of this writing, you may visit this website for more information on how to donate umbilical cord blood through the Cord for Life Program of Cryobanks International.

https://cordforlife.lifeforcecryobanks.com/public-donation.html

Looking back, I wholeheartedly acknowledge that I wasn't paying enough attention to my mother's medical care with the absolute precision that I ordinarily would have under regular circumstances.

How could I possibly be expected to engage in an epistemological debate about rationale for different variations on cancer treatment when I was learning to be a new mother at the same time?

I came home from the hospital, recovering from a caesarian section, still learning to nurse my infant, wondering how anyone could possibly have more than one child when having one was so incredibly life altering. Little did I know what was yet to come. While my parents quietly and desperately fought to regain their normal lives post-transplant, my husband and I struggled through all the trials and tribulations that new parents do. Not once since the day before the baby was born have I actually layed in bed watching Friends and Sex in the City reruns.

IF THERE IS ANYTHING I CAN DO...

If there is *anything* you can do? You mean, at your convenience of course. Because if it's an inconvenience to you, then forget about it, all bets are off. There is only one person on the face of the earth who will do something for you that is an inconvenience and that is your own mother. A mother will do just about anything for her child, whether an infant or an adult. Everyone else is subject to doing things at their own convenience. Even the most well intentioned people do this, perhaps unknowingly, but they do it anyway.

Someone close to me calls at 4:00 pm on the second day I was home from the hospital after having a C-section with my *second* child and says "is there anything I can do?" yes, do you think you could pick up some maxi pads for me? Sure, but I'm meeting a friend for dinner tonight, so I'll bring them by after that." Um, sure, no problem, but why then did you ask if there was anything you could do? I should be grateful enough that she is going to pick them up for me, but in the meantime, maybe I'll just wad up some toilet paper and stick it in my underwear. I can barely move from my bed anyway, so it's not a problem if I get blood stains on my sheets because it's not like anyone else is going to see them or wash them for me anyway. Did I mention I could just use a glass of water? At this point I don't even care if it's brown tap water from the bathroom, my throat is so dry and I can't move; I just need a glass of water. I'll deal with the bloody sheets later.

By now it is the spring of 2008; my mom went back in the hospital in December due to complications from the bone marrow transplant. The physicians warned us about the "complications" and we followed their instructions to a T, yet her health was quickly deteriorating while I tried desperately to remain strong and centered with a newborn and a 14 month old. What people need, especially from their medical practitioners is nutritional literacy, not a schedule of warnings about the toxicity of the 15 different medications that were prescribed to overcome the transplant. Even if we do need that, okay, we do, but we need it in conjunction with the right information about diet and disease.

Children test our resolve. Day in and day out, by the hour, by the minute. Children bring us more joy than we ever thought possible, while at the same time, driving us over the edge of sanity. People have different ways of staying tolerant, and some are much better at it than others.

89

How do we better cope with our own children when we're faced with the adversities of life? Or worse, grief and loss? The answer lies within. Deep within. Contemplate, read, process, understand, and in the case of what I did: embrace the parallel that running has to offer.

Runners Never Stop Running

It's been said that runs don't end with a particular race. It's been said that life is about the journey, not the destination. If you really take a moment to reach inside your soul, you will probably find that you are the only one who controls the type of life you lead. We all know people who are happy all the time. Are they on drugs? How are they happy all the time? Don't they have problems like the rest of us? Real big problems, like dealing with a cancer diagnosis or finding a way to pay the mortgage next month, putting food on the table, and competing for a job when 25 other over qualified applicants have also applied for the same position.

There are a million reasons to be upset. Your car needs to be fixed. Your boss stole your idea. Your neighbor's dog crapped on your lawn for the 10th time this week. Your 2-year old made a spectacle in Target and complete strangers looked at you like you were the worst parent in the world. Did I mention the screaming child arched her back when you tried to strap her in the car seat or the fact that you discovered some small item in her hand when you got home which you do not remember placing on the belt at the register so quite possibly you discover that you must be a shoplifter? Maybe you got signals crossed with your husband this morning because you just got home from a run and he was on his way out the door when you told him *not to use the ATM card* because we have exactly to the cent enough money to cover an electronic bill that is being drafted today, yet his car has had the empty light on for the past 2 days so he needed gas and used the ATM card because he didn't hear you. Now, not only is there a deficit in your bank account for the price of the gas, but there is a $30.00 insufficient funds fee from the bank as well. Sweet. These things happen to everyone. The sooner you realize that everyone else in the world has challenges to work through just like you do, the easier life will be. It's not a reason to not eat healthy.

Some people worry too much about what other people think. Luckily we runners share something in common, and it's usually that we concern ourselves with our own self and don't really care too much about what other people think of us. I can remember when a friend of mine first started running with me. We couldn't run on a certain road because she had this fear that people driving by would see her running and reach the conclusion that she was running too slow. Well, I don't know about you, but when I'm driving in my car and I see a runner, I usually can't even judge how fast or slow the person is running, nor do I care, nor do I even have time to judge whether that might be someone I know. I mean, most of us are in the car driving with the intention of going somewhere. Does anybody really have the time to put that much thought into who is running on the side of the road? I mean seriously, if you see me running and I don't wave to you, it's not your fault; I just wasn't paying attention to you. My friend eventually got over her fear of running on that road, but the point is, nobody cares how fast you're running or what you're wearing, or how far you went. Once you come to the realization that you are the only person putting that pressure on yourself you will be better off. The fact that you are out there, exercising, becoming physically fit, breathing in the fresh air, not caring what anybody thinks of you; that is testament that you are one step closer to being at peace with your inner-self.

The moral of the story here is that nobody cares what you put in your cart at the grocery store except you. Nobody cares what is inside your child's lunchbox except you. Whether you are in the midst of dealing with a disease in the family or in the midst of raising a family, a run or walk can help you get back to what is most important. It can help you enjoy the world around us; help you see beauty in yourself and in others. It can help you embrace the happiness of childhood, be content, be silly, be grounded. It's a place where you can lose yourself in your own thoughts, or surround yourself with people to talk to. Running can become an addiction to those endorphins in your brain that make you happy. You can run for yourself, run for a cause, run with a friend, or find a friend. Running was my way of coping with the series of life changing circumstances....my two children, born just shy of 14 months apart, and the death of my mother, when my youngest was just 2 weeks old.

Running forced me to focus on nutrition, specifically, how to fuel my body for a marathon, a distance of 26.2 miles. I read a lot of literature about endurance athletes while training for my first marathon, and even spoke to dozens of people who completed the distance many times over. Just like in the hospital setting, not once did I hear about a whole-foods, plant-based diet being the primary focus of optimal health or performance. Instead, most of the information pointed to protein. What I found from my own experience is that eating too much protein before intense exercise results in muscle cramping. You don't need a degree in biochemistry to know that protein requires a lot more effort, thus, fluid, for the body to metabolize than plants; further, cramping occurs in runners when the body is not properly hydrated. Have you ever run a marathon and wondered why so many people are walking at mile 20 instead of running? Hello, you've got 6 more miles to go! If you walk now, it may take you hours to finish, if you finish at all!

I learned that even professional athletes rely on misguided information, they don't realize that they could actually perform better if they significantly cut back on animal protein and switched to a plant-based diet. The reason is because obtaining the optimal amount of protein, fiber, and other essential nutrients from plants (rather than an excess of protein from meats and animal based products) actually allows the body to recover faster from a difficult and strenuous workout. Since the body can recover faster, the athlete can move on to another difficult workout sooner, thus building more strength and endurance. Therefore, it is the whole foods that actually provide the platform on which long-term, sustainable health and vitality is gained, not the simple sugars that are touted as beneficial for the short term.

So many runners I know believe that athletes need a snack shortly before they run a distance, but then they look to the protein bar. Here is the problem with the protein bar: the rise in cortisol level that accompanies a short term energy snack like a protein bar always results in fatigue. In actuality, any kind of stimulation that produces short-term energy (coffee, all snacks made with refined sugars or simple carbs) is always followed by fatigue.[25] Would you consider eating a candy bar before running 26.2 miles as healthy? I didn't think so. Don't be fooled once again by the marketing tactics...those clever folks want you to believe that the product contains the slow release of energy, which is false. If you carefully consider the nutrient label, you'll find that the protein bar is nothing but a glorified candy bar.

Don't even get me started on sports drinks. What you need to know about sports drinks is that unless you are a seasoned athlete completing an extraordinary endurance event, your body does not need all of the additives (read chemicals) in a sports drink. Remember the large advertising budgets of the manufacturers?

We have sexy athletes and celebrities doing commercials that sell these sugary energy drinks. A subconscious connection is made with an unknowing consumer on a very sensual level; by making a visual connection, for just a few seconds, the typical consumer believes, somehow, because that athlete or celebrity is glamorized in their sport that they too participate in that sport, so it must be good for them too.

WHY COW'S MILK IS FOR BABY COWS AND NOT BABY HUMAN BEINGS...

Breastfeeding an infant is one of the hardest things to learn how to do, but once you master it, it is the easiest, least expensive, most convenient, and most nutritious way to feed your baby. Experts in the medical arena as well as health-related seminars and booklets produced by government agencies on nursing infants, all emphatically point to this conclusion, but once again convenience in America wins out over wellness and the mainstream population at large remains in the dark about the real importance of feeding your infant mother's milk over that which is meant for a baby cow.

My experience with this fundamentally important nutritional issue started in the hospital, with the first shift change of the nursing staff after my baby was born. For starters, every nurse thinks that her way of breastfeeding is the correct way, and heaven forbid you don't do it *her* way, then you are doing it the wrong way. The first nurse I encountered was of course the one I trusted first. When I came out of my laboring experience, my hands were still shaking, for that matter my whole body was still shaking...to the point that I couldn't even hold my baby because I was so heavily medicated by pharmaceutical drugs.

So new mothers will find this section entertaining, and everyone else, well, you might just be taken back to that time when you'll remember this amusing and very real experience.

The nurse holds the baby to my breast and the baby's head "shakes" from side to side. It was pretty funny, here I was laying helpless and my new baby's lips are trying desperately to get on my nipple and the nurse is saying "obviously this isn't working" well no kidding sister, you're not holding the baby in the right position and I sure can't get a good grip on her. So she says "let's try this nipple guard" and proceeds to put this plastic thing over my nipple. It looks like a clear pacifier and I'm wondering how my baby is supposed to suck on my breast through this thing and actually get the milk. It looks like it should fit on a bottle, but instead she puts it on my breast like the breast is a bottle. The actual tip has like 5 holes in it and it's huge. I wonder if my nipple is supposed to fit into it, because it sure doesn't look like it will. The truth? By the time you become expert at breastfeeding, your nipples actually get so darn big and puffed up, like the size of your pinky finger from the last knuckle to the tip. You might as well be a porn star. Does a nipple really get that big? If you're breastfeeding it does. Oh, and another thing.....you know how regular baby bottle "nipples" have one hole at the tip? Well, if you're breastfeeding, your nipples have like 20 holes that the milk streams out of. Weird. I didn't find this out until I used the electric breast pump for the first time and was in awe of how many little tiny holes the milk came out of. They are not in the areola, even though all the books say to get as much of the areola into the baby's mouth as possible. The milk comes only through the tip. It actually gets as big as a bottle nipple. Ah, so that's why the make the bottle nipples so large.

Anyway, back to the plastic device that is supposed to be helping me breastfeed for the very first time ever. It's totally not working. The nurse takes the baby away and says "you can try again later". Um, ok, does the baby need to eat or not? I guess not. The truth is, the baby really doesn't need to eat immediately because the baby doesn't recognize the feeling of hunger yet. So you have a short window of opportunity to recover from the headache of labor. Gosh women are vain sometimes, but yes, I just told you that story because it's relatively amusing to any mother who has been there, done that.

A few hours later it's time to try again, only this time, I'm in the post-partum room and feeling a little bit better. So by now a new set of nurses hustle the baby into the room (she was in the nursery while they moved me from the labor room to another room) and say "she needs to eat" so they put her on my belly. I'm like, um, uh, ok, and the baby's head shaking the same way as it was before. I hold her head with my hand and try to get her mouth around the areola like I learned in the classes. Finally she "latches on" and appears to be sucking. It doesn't hurt. The first few tries, the baby puts her mouth on you and sucks, but doesn't "latch". So, how do you get her to latch? She has to have the actual tip of the nipple right smack in the middle of her throat and you do that by smashing the baby's nose into the top of the breast. The lactation consultants will tell you that babies only know how to breathe through their nose, so even if the nose is pressed right up against, the little corners of their nostril will allow them to breathe. The baby has a very powerful and forceful suck, I'm talking piranha. *I'm not kidding.* Furthermore, a nursing infant leans toward and sucks anything that his or her mouth gets close to...including arms, shoulders, and anybody else that holds him or her gets treated as if their breast will produce milk too. It's funny how after a while you notice who is familiar with breastfeeding and who is not because all exclusive breastfed babies have the reflex of turning toward the breast when they are "cradled" or held in the baby position by anyone, including men. Similar to the seasoned moms, most women just laugh and say "those don't work anymore" or just hand the baby back and say "I think she's hungry."

So, okay, back to the first feeding...due to the piranha nature of the baby, the areola turn black and blue quite easily, the nurses call this bruising. "Oh, you are so bruised" well yes smarty pants, if you would let me get to know my baby and do this my own way instead of trying to make me try it your way then that might help. This is a big discouraging point for a brand new nursing mother, especially one whose own mother is too far away to provide support. Your nipples are black and blue and they might even be cracking and bleeding and getting so chapped that you are about to give up. I finally Googled sore nipples, and after trying not to look like a weirdo when porn sites came up, I found sites that suggested heat, ice, and lanolin. Ugh. How do I know if the baby is getting enough to eat? I was charting like crazy. Every hour, how long did she eat? What time did she start? Well, this wasn't working because she would start and then stop, fall asleep, or be hungry at will. They say "feed her every 2-4 hours" that doesn't make any sense because in reality, it seemed my baby was hungry every 15 minutes! Why? She would fall asleep just when I thought we got the hang of it. Then she would all of a sudden wake up and shriek as if somebody just smacked her face or something. Thank goodness for Google. What did anyone do before the internet? I really need my mom. God I miss her. Why is the baby screaming like a nut? What the hell did I do or didn't I do that I'm supposed to be doing?

It turns out that the babies stomach is so tiny, that she eats like a tablespoon of breastmilk when she's a day old. Yes, a tablespoon. That's all she needs. Innately, a newborn infant has the ability to moderate her own satiety?

SATIETY

How do we conceptualize satiety and the impossible complexity of the feeding the proper amount to the human body? The thought came into the spotlight a few years later when my 4 year old asked for a "snack" an hour after eating breakfast. Could he still be hungry? It is important to know that food-like products are designed around the fact that your child *should be hungry* an hour after you feed them. That is not what nature intended.[26] The American public has been led to believe that we should eat every 2-3 hours, we consistently have snacks all day long instead of eating 3 meals a day. Nutrition experts and weight loss "programs" are telling us to snack and graze, and it's rubbing off on our children. The fact is, if we eat the foods we're supposed to be eating, with naturally occurring fiber and complex carbohydrates instead of refined simple sugars, then our body is not hungry an hour after we eat. That is the concept of "satiety". Realize then that if you learn how to eat properly you will never have to count calories, because calories don't count. Period. Why are we hungry an hour after we eat? Because we're eating the wrong foods. Remember back to Chapter 2: refined foods include any food that is not a whole food. By eating refined foods, our blood insulin is tricked. It happens during digestion, whether you believe you can control it or not...you simply cannot control it unless you stop eating the wrong kinds of foods.

What do you do? First of all, realize that about 90% of the cereals in the cereal aisle in your grocery store (as well as 90% of the bread in the bread aisle) contain the wrong ingredients. If "Enriched Wheat Flour" is the first ingredient, that is the first problem. There are two easy options to help you make the right choice at breakfast: Whole oats or sprouted grain breads. Eating unsweetened, rolled oats, (not the sweetened kind) guarantees you are eating a whole grain. Remember back to Jeff Novick's rules for ingredient labels. If the ingredient label contains the words "cracked and stone ground" followed by a grain as the first ingredient, that will help ensure you are making the right choice. Be sure to use a dairy alternative such as Rice Milk or Almond Milk (I like unsweetened) because otherwise you expose yourself to the harmful animal casein in dairy milk. (Yogurt comes in non-dairy alternatives too, my favorite almond milk yogurt is by a brand called Amande). Whole grains in combination with fresh fruit of any kind are among the best ways to reduce hunger for hours.

A mother's milk, we know, is the perfect food for a baby. Perfect because it is specifically formulated for baby, obviously she's been eating what you've been eating for nearly 10 months, so she's used to your diet. Obviously an infant practically doubles in size during the first year of his or her life. Think about that for a minute. Consuming only a mother's milk, and no food, a baby *doubles in size.* At no other time in life will a human being double in size in such a short amount of time. Further, a breastfed baby, 9 times out of 10, will not have any issues with being allergic or having upset stomach or gas when exclusively breast fed because again, she's used to your diet. I learned in my breastfeeding class that there are literally hundreds of nutrients in breast milk, and even the DHA and AHA fortified formulas can only replicate like 30 of those nutrients. The exact same concept applies to the foods we consume today. Plant-based foods, in their whole form, contain vitamins, minerals, and phytochemicals that synergistically cause enzymatic reactions during digestion that a supplement simply cannot replicate. In fact, foods in the Western or American diet are deficient in so many nutrients that our bodies have sustained significant damage from eating these disease-promoting foods. Since breast milk is more easily digested than formula, it goes through the babies system much faster. That is why breastfed babies need to eat every 2 hours instead of every 4 like bottle-fed babies. Don't fret, as the baby grows and eats more, the baby does not have to eat every 2 hours. Let's take a look at dairy…cow's milk. Assuming your child is over the age of 2, would you feed him or her a glass of milk that contains over 100 different types of puss? That's right, I said 100 types of puss in one glass of milk.[27] That is disgusting.

The American Academy of Pediatrics, who the public looks to for recommendations for about nutritional and medical information for infants and children is convinced enough to suggest that infants should not be exposed to cow's milk for the first two years of life, but has not yet acknowledged that children should stop drinking cow's milk after the age of 2. In fact, for babies weaned off the breast before age 2, they issued a statement in July 2008 recommending that children with a family history of obesity be given 2% milk (after they are weaned until age 2). The group then recommended that after age 2, the kids be placed on 1% fat milk.[11]

CAN THE BABY EAT SCABS?

So, for the moms, and anyone else who is amused by the details of nursing an infant…the bruising, aching, pain, and blood…can the baby eat the scabs? Yes, eat up. In other words, blister right on through it because it sure hurts you more than it hurts the baby. So by now the nipples are burning, they are on fire, not only while the baby is eating but all the stinking time. It seriously feels like the baby actually bit the nipple off and left the wound open and inflamed for all the world to see. Ouch! This fucking hurts!

This is the first of many sacrifices you will make for your precious little one. How do you really deal? I'm barely able to get up out of bed, but I'm at the pharmacy searching the baby aisle for the latest and greatest in nipple treatment. The lanolin is not doing anything for me. The gel things feel pretty good for right after the feeding, but then you have to wipe the gel off before the next feeding. So, basically what happens is you feed the baby, put the gels on, just when you doze off to get 10 minutes rest, the baby is hungry again and you're yelling at your husband to bring you a warm cloth to wipe the gel off the nipple so the baby doesn't get poisoned. In the time it takes him to walk from the bathroom to your bed (remember, you're still in your hospital room) the cloth gets cold and hurts. Why can't he make it hot so it's warm by the time he gets it to me? Then, the wipe, OUCH! Then the baby is trying to latch, OUCH!! So you rush to all 3 drugstores that are within a mile of your house and buy them out of the gel pads. Why don't these idiots carry more gel pads? Why are there only 3 boxes on the shelf but there are 20 boxes of disposable breast pads? Those don't help my sore nipples at all. They do serve an important purpose though, I just haven't gotten there yet because the baby is still only one day old.

So the gel pads provide temporary relief, and I mean temporary since the feedings occur every 2 hours. The nurses give this approximate time frame of 2 hours, except they are counting the 2 hours from the beginning of the feeding. So, if you're like all new breastfeeding mothers then you know that the baby will stay on one breast for 45 minutes and you're wondering whether this is totally normal. I mean, as soon as the precious thing is finished, it's nearly time to begin another feeding. Well, the truth? Feed the baby when the baby is hungry, and only leave the baby on one breast for a maximum of 20 minutes. Believe me when I tell you that once the baby figures out how to eat, he or she will be able to consume the meal in 10 minutes flat and be done.

You'll know when the baby has learned this because of what I call the "drunken baby" syndrome. The baby latches on, take a few sucks to start the flow of milk, then takes these long sips...slurrrrrrrrrrrrrrrrrrp, slurrrrrrrrrrrrp, for like 40 counts. You know...you count 1 for each long slurp and eventually there are so many you lose your count. Seriously, did you count the slurps too? Then the sucking slows down. The baby either falls off the nipple asleep or you can just barely give a small tug out of the baby's mouth. Don't by any means try to tug out of the baby's mouth while the baby is in the process of sucking or you will feel the biggest ouch of your life. You can only, I repeat, only do this when the baby is in the "drunken" state. How do you know when your baby is in the drunken state? Well, the baby is pretty much lethargic, indifferent to anything that is going on around him, and looks like he could be passed out. He is extremely heavy, like dead weight in your arms, and very, very content. Ahhhh, the true sign of a belly full of mother's milk. This of course is the best time to cuddle your little price or princess and then put him or her down in bed to sleep. Holding your drunken baby makes all the nipple soreness seem to melt away. Oh yes, and breastfeeding pays dividends later. Big dividends. Ear infection? What's that? Exactly. Do it, you'll be glad you did.

Do you get that satisfying, content, "baby drunk" feeling after eating Thanksgiving dinner? Or is your dinner so delicious that you force yourself to consume large amounts of food so that you have to open the button on your pants and then lay on the couch for the rest of the day? Exactly. This is what mainstream Americans do...they use food as a source of contentment rather than nourishment. I'm not suggesting food should not be a matter of contentment, but let's find the happy medium so we can be content and healthy at the same time.

Maybe you celebrate holidays with certain foods because you've done that for the past few decades, but if you just step back and consider for a moment that the celebration is more about the people gathering together, and less about the jar of canned green beans, then maybe, just maybe, you can make some small changes and move you toward better health.

Why do people overeat one meal and then spend the next 5 days consuming nothing but a "protein shake" instead of enjoying the meal preparation and experience of flavor combinations that tantalize the palate? You've surely heard about that person at your office who eats the cake and then talks about how guilty they feel for the next 3 days and how they should not have eaten that second serving.

Cuisine has undergone an exceptional transformation over the past few decades with the availability of global ingredients, yet instead of considering the appropriateness of meal preparation that is based on such factors as weather or occasion, Americans still choose convenience. Because it's not widely known that what we eat directly impacts not only how we feel on any given day, but drastically alters chronic disease, we hardly give it a second thought. Finally science and medicine are coming full circle, and people are recognizing that what we have done to the environment is already having a significant impact on disease, as the familiar American jingle dictates: from the oceans to the prairies to the mountains white with snow. From our over-fished oceans to the depleted soils to the deficiency that exists in a country of excess, the only way to move forward is to understand the connection between what we eat and the essence of life. The deeper your understanding of these connections, the greater your ability to achieve peace and happiness.

I obviously believe overall wellness is deeply rooted in nutrition, but that is not the only factor. We know that exercise and sleep fit into the mix, but there is another element. It's an element that has been studied for hundreds of years in the East but one that isn't given much consideration in our Western society today, and that is the spiritual component. I'm not a particularly spiritual person, even though I was raised Catholic. Whatever religious beliefs you have or have not is not the point; the fundamental connection lies in one's ability to manage the stresses of everyday life and achieve a level of relaxation through things like self-reflection, spiritual connectedness, massage, or appreciation of simplicity.

When you think about it, doing something as simple as planting a garden in your back yard offers all of the aforementioned associations. You create life and watch it grow, teach a child lessons of patience and gratitude, harvest your bounty, cook the meal together as a family, and then taste the flavor combinations of vegetables and herbs while savoring the essence of that moment. Gather with friends and family, discuss the day's events around a table filled with laughter and smiles. Now, you've engaged in something important and significant, you've created memories that will last a lifetime. You've ensured that your food is free of chemical contaminants and enjoyed what nature has to offer, and it's all because you planted a garden. It's time to trade the garden for the jar of cranberry sauce.

So...the pharmacy: why on earth are there are a million boxes of disposable breast pads? The reality is, once you get past the sore nipple syndrome of the first few days, the only thing you need is the disposable pads. Why? I was wondering the same myself until I realized all this business about the "let down" reflex. When your precious baby is doing the 40 long sucks on one breast, the other one is leaking out some serious milk. You can't just sit there or your shirt will be drenched. It actually looks like somebody poured a glass of milk on your shirt. So, you wear the nursing bra, with the disposable breast pad on the opposite side of where the baby is currently eating. Your other breast will leak out a river of milk and if you don't have anything there to trap it, you will be literally wearing a soaking wet shirt. I'm not talking about a little bit of wetness, I'm talking about soaking wet like you just pulled this shirt out of the washing machine and forgot to put it into the dryer before you put it on. So, I went through probably a box of breast pads a week for the entire amount of time I nursed. This now explains why there are so many boxes of disposable ones at the pharmacy.

Now that we've covered babies and milk, what about those commercials on television that suggest that women need more calcium in their diet to help prevent osteoporosis?

OSTEOPEROSIS

Here is some food for thought: While milk does contain calcium and protein, that doesn't mean it reduces the risk of osteoporosis as you age. In fact, many research studies have shown that it does the exact opposite! Studies show an important connection between intake of calcium and animal protein pointing toward a higher risk of osteoporosis, not lower. Researchers found that the protein in milk can actually weaken bones, especially when not enough "protective" plant-based foods are consumed.

In a study published in the *American Journal of Clinical Nutrition*[12], researchers followed 1035 white women older than 65 and recorded their protein intake and bone mineral density. It was reported that "an increase in vegetable protein intake and a decrease in animal protein intake may decrease bone loss and the risk of hip fracture." Another study from the *Journals of Gerontology*[13] looked at hip fracture, and mimicked the findings of the first study. A direct link to animal protein intake and compromised bone integrity was found.

Most studies depend on participants' self reporting, their ability to recall what they ate and when. I don't know about you, but I can barely remember what I had for breakfast 3 days ago, let alone 3 weeks ago. But what I can tell you for certain is that I am not worried about trying to add more calcium to my diet.

Some notes I took on a lecture I heard by Colin Campbell can explain better than I can the difference between animal protein and plant protein with regard to how vitamins and minerals (such as calcium) are digested:

> The amino acids present in animal protein, as opposed to the amino acids present in plant protein, get metabolized, altered, excreted, and changed during digestion. Consuming animal protein produces an acid-like condition in the human body which is not natural and not tolerated well. Our bodies are incredibly complex, so all systems work together to reduce the acidity. Essentially, to reduce the acidity, the body draws on the metabolized calcium that is present in the bones. The acid in the body that is being neutralized by the calcium present in the bones is then lost in the urine; this is the process that weakens the bones. All because of the animal protein consumption. So the moral of the story? Don't worry so much about drinking milk or taking a calcium supplement…instead, eat more vegetables so that the calcium your body

produces naturally isn't used up to metabolize the meat that you eat and the milk that you drink.

Still need more evidence? How about as far back as 2005 when a review published in *Pediatrics* showed that milk consumption does not improve bone integrity in children.[18] Similarly, the Harvard Nurses' Health Study, one of the largest and most well know studies on the relationship between cancer and diet which followed more than 72,000 women for 18 years, showed no protective effect of increased milk consumption.[19]

WHAT IS THIS SAYING
ABOUT AMERICAN CULTURE?

For one, the greed of an entire society, an entire healthcare system, an entire industrialized food system continues to manifest most notably in our hospitals, in our military, and for goodness sake in our own children's school lunch system. We complain that nobody is doing anything about it, place blame on the President or on "the system" itself. Instead, we need to start in our own homes; first by understanding how and why the corruption exists. Then, we need to remember that we, the American citizens, control supply and demand. We are the consumers, you and me. If you don't buy the milk laced with casein, hormones and antibiotics, then the government will be forced to evaluate programs that make it easier for organic farmers to benefit, and harder for those who keep turning to antibiotics, pesticides, herbicides and fungicides to keep ruling our food system.

I don't know about you, but this is pretty compelling evidence; it is why I don't serve cow's milk to my children. It's a tough call, because in reality what are kids supposed to drink? Water, yes, but they do need sometimes need a little something different, especially on a really hot day in the middle of the summer when the temperature and humidity are at the highest. It's not that I think fruit "juice" is all that bad, the problem is the amount of excess sugar and artificial chemicals that are added into the box juices. Even dentists recommend against serving fruit juice to children because it significantly increases the risk of tooth decay.

Here are some tips on juice: The first thing you might want to do on a hot day is slice up a bowl of oranges. Then you can be 100% sure that you're not getting anything artificial or any added sugar. Believe me, when it's that hot and oranges are all you have to offer, your children will eat them, or at least suck the juice out of them! I've made it a habit to bring a bowl of sliced fresh oranges, pineapple, or watermelon anytime I attend an outdoor summer function with my kids. I find that because kids are highly influenced by what others do, if at least one child is eating the fresh fruit then the others will follow suit.

Other recommendations: bring frozen grapes or make fruit kabobs. These are all ways you can give children the fresh fruit instead of processed juices. I also like to squeeze my own lemonade. When I'm making fresh lemonade, the only ingredients are water, lemon juice and a touch of sugar. I actually make the simple syrup, dissolve a bit of sugar in water over moderate heat, to just sweeten it up slightly. While yes, this is added sugar, I can monitor exactly how much added sugar. A much better alternative to buying premade lemonade which can contain up to 8 teaspoons of sugar per serving. Yikes. If you absolutely must give your children juice in a "box" or "pouch" I like the Honest Kids brand, from the makers of Honest Tea Inc., Bethesda, Maryland. This juice is certified organic and contains myriad less sugar and added artificial ingredients that all of the other alternatives on your grocery store shelf.

Becoming a parent was a major contributing factor in furthering my obsession with proper nutrition, not only because it changes every facet of your life beginning with the moment a child is born, but because of the sheer responsibility involved in raising a tiny human being to become a happy, healthy, contributing member of society. Suddenly, the way I eat becomes not only about my husband and me, but about falling in love all over again...with the tiny little person that we both created. Any parent knows that feeling cannot be understood by anyone until they actually produce a child of their own. Even people who love babies and children just cannot fully comprehend the magnitude of child birth until it happens. Everything you do from that moment on becomes about the baby...and that's okay. Just remember, your husband loved you before he loved the baby, so keep in mind that change happens and you just have to be flexible and go with it. I think I gained a new kind of love for my husband after the whole baby experience. Of course I still love him as much as I did before the baby(ies) came, but now, I love *the way he loves our children,* and that makes me love him even more.

For that, I am truly grateful.

Part IV
Scientifically Speaking

Part IV
Scientifically Speaking

Chapter 9: Food Combinations

Mmm. Foodies know that certain combinations are pure indulgence. Classic combinations include summer ripe tomato with fresh basil, oranges and figs in the fall, or apples and cinnamon with fresh thyme and blueberry sauce. What we sometimes don't realize is that food combinations are not only tasty on the palate, they serve an incredibly complex biochemical purpose when combined properly. On the other side of the equation, certain combinations can also be extremely taxing on our digestive system. Ahem, bacon and eggs.

Whole Foods, Plant-Based Nutrition

I don't particularly like the term "vegan". I think it has underlying connotations and associations with the stereotypical 1960s tree-hugger types who are pure animal rights activists. Don't get me wrong, I mean, I respect animals, but I have also been known to wear snakeskin pumps and carry a leather handbag. I have not been vegan my entire life, and don't be surprised, as I mentioned earlier, if you see me allowing my children to eat ice cream once or twice a year (we'll be under the boardwalk). That is the key, I am human and I make an exception once or twice a year, not once or twice a week! This is precisely why I like to use the term "plant-based" and associate my way of eating as a diet of *primarily* whole-foods, plant-based nutrition rather than "vegan."

Just look at the cookbooks out there on the market; people claim to be vegan, and then the recipe includes oil, soy, and a partially hydrogenated cheese substitute. Sure, you can find cookbooks that replicate an old favorite such as "Pasta with Meat-Less Balls". Really? Meatless balls? What are those balls made out of? You guessed it: processed soy, hydrogenated oils, and other chemicals which are actually more harmful to consume on an ongoing basis than actually having one serving of meat once per year. To make a plant-based diet work, you have to stick to the beauty of the plant foods and stop trying to replicate traditional recipes with shady substitutions. Certainly, if you are in danger of any vascular diseases, you need to really focus on eliminating all of the harmful products, including "vegan" versions which can still contain hydrogenated oils and artificial sweeteners, including non-natural ones like Agave. Let's get over the "junk" vegan and move toward whole foods, plant-based nutrition.

More on Agave you ask? This sweetener is a favorite among vegans, prized for its "low glycemic" miracle, but what you may not know is that agave "nectar" or agave "syrup" is produced through a highly chemical process using genetically modified enzymes, caustic acids, and filtration chemicals. [29]

Agave is devoid of virtually all nutrient value and actually has a higher fructose content than most commercial sweeteners (ranging from 55-97% depending on the brand), which is much higher than high fructose corn syrup which averages about 55%. Agave's high fructose levels go directly to the liver, where it is stored as blood fat (also known as triglycerides) which increases heart disease risk factors. These high fructose levels also contribute to insulin resistance as well as nonalcoholic fatty liver disease. So if you are substituting Agave for sweetener, make sure you do it in moderation. The better bet is to use a naturally occurring sweetener like raw honey or organic maple syrup. Some vegans do not consume honey because it comes from a bee which they consider an animal. Remember, I'm plant-based, not vegan, so I'm okay with honey.

While we generally strive to make healthy choices, once you dive into the world of nutrition, you realize it opens the door to so many more questions. Before I cover more on food combinations, I thought it would be important to discuss the role vitamins play in the process.

The ingestion of large amounts of specific nutrients, in the form of vitamins, actually interferes with absorption and metabolism of other nutrients in the body.

Vitamins

There is a lot of conflicting information out there, and I think most of it stems from the industries with the deepest pockets because as you already know, they have the ability to influence what regular people believe. Unfortunately the lonely kohlrabi sits on a cold, misty shelf and gets overlooked because nobody has heard of it while the Dora the Explorer fruit-like snack (that really has no fruit what so ever in it) garners the most attention, further exasperated with prime low level shelf space so the toddler can grab it and throw a temper tantrum if he doesn't get it, which then causes the parent to either 1. look like a parent who cannot control their toddler or 2. buy the box of processed non-food so the toddler stops screaming. Since society is so politically correct of late, most people buy the box of junk food because it's easier.

Why can't someone invent a Dora the Explorer wrapper
for bananas?

The point is, most people are highly influenced by their visual senses, and we all know a picture is worth a thousand words. It is so important to get past the marketing budgets and think critically about what we are consuming from the perspective of overall wellness, and this goes for vitamins too. There are simply foods that have had vitamin or mineral supplements added in, sometimes called "fortified". Often, this is done because they have been processed, and some of the natural vitamins and minerals have been removed during the refining process, such as with white rice compared to brown rice. Most bread, for example, is processed, and as such requires fortification to sell better because the packaging can then claim "high in calcium" or "contains vitamin D". You simply cannot replace a food with a supplement.

Here is another example: enter marketing budgets from sources such as the largest pharmaceutical companies. For the average person, I think this is especially evident in the pharmaceutical commercials we see on television now more than ever before. In order to evaluate the "design" (of a scientific study) for the average person, he or she might consider the commercial that says something like "Ask your doctor if this drug is right for you." (You might have 100 different side effects, but ask anyway....) I think now society is finally at the point where ordinary people are finally starting to question the validity of some of these claims. While the commercial isn't the scientific paper, for the average person it sort of represents the claim that the drug company is making. It's important to help people realize that the claim (the commercial) is basically just one viewpoint (ie: the single nutrient/pill that could potentially produce adverse effects on other systems in the body) and not necessarily indicative of a way to promote a healthy lifestyle.

People view vitamins as a way to help supplement the foods they eat and protect against disease or nutrient deficiencies. However, it is not the vitamin that protects from disease, it is the nutrients contained in the vitamin that helps build up our immune system so that our own body can protect us from disease. By consuming the vitamin, we overlook the thousands of phytochemicals in the whole plant foods, which in reality is what provides substantially more health benefits than a supplement ever could.

Here are a few commonly known[28] examples:

•Calcium inhibits heme and nonheme iron absorption

•Iron inhibits zinc absorption

•Zinc inhibits copper absorption

•Vitamin E antagonizes vitamin K action

•Vitamin E may decrease levels of circulating prothrombin

•Polyphenols from tea extracts inhibited nonheme iron absorption

•Foliate interferes with vitamin B12 metabolism

•Beta carotene can inhibit lutein absorption when they are given together as supplements, although not when lutein and beta carotene are given together in the form of genetically selected yellow carrots

•Supplementing with relatively high doses of {alpha}-tocopherol decreases plasma levels of {Delta}- and {gamma}-tocopherol

The truth? I really don't even know what some of that means; I had to google the word prothrombin* but what I can say is that vitamin supplements fit into that confusing biochemistry and clearly alter the natural metabolism of your food. Have you ever read the label of a vitamin bottle or pharmaceutical drug that warns against taking it with milk or certain other foods? The interaction of the pill and those foods during digestion are precisely what the warning is about. Experts agree that additional consideration is exasperated even further when considering questions of physiological need, nutrient balance, timing, duration, dosage and product-related issues such as purity, potency, contamination, industrial processing, and additives.

There is that word again, additives. As I was writing this portion of the book another report came out about hypertension in children. The study[10] analyzed more than 6,000 medical records of children, ages 12 through 17, from a national databank, the scientists found that teenagers with abnormally high levels of uric acid in their blood were, on average, twice as likely to have high blood pressure as those with normal levels. The investigators also warned that a single episode of high blood pressure does not necessarily mean hypertension, but that elevated blood pressure on three consecutive visits to the doctor is classified as hypertension. The lead investigator, Lauren Loeffler, M.D., M.H.S., a nephrologist at Johns Hopkins Children's Center says: "High blood pressure is no longer an adult disease and is an increasingly common problem among children today. These findings illuminate one potential pathway in the development of hypertension in the young and suggests a way for detection and treatment."

---

*prothrombin: measure of the extrinsic pathway of coagulation (blood clotting), used to determine the clotting tendency in the liver

So like we said before, children are being diagnosed earlier and prescribed medication for the rest of their lives? How is this better? The other childhood disease we also spoke of earlier, Type 1 diabetes, is increasing at an alarming rate of 3% per year.[14] It was found that the children who were genetically susceptible to type 1 diabetes, when fed cow's milk, actually upped their risk of the disease by 11-13 times what it would otherwise have been in the children who were not genetically predisposed.[15]

Remember nutrient balance is critical to our biochemical function and just like milk, vitamins initiate a sequence of biochemical adjustments in our body to maintain a requisite internal equilibrium, just like pharmaceutical medications do. I've read some books that point toward vitamins as being something people who can afford to buy them do to sustain their health. While this may be true from an observational standpoint, what you should take away from that is the idea that healthy people tend to be healthy because of their diet and exercise program, not because of their vitamin intake.

Here is some additional information and online resources (current as of the time this book was published) about vitamin supplementation:

•Vitamin Overdosing in Preschool Age Children: A study of 1,847 preschoolers in Belgium, published in the journal Appetite (2010), suggested that both supplement users and those who didn't take them were often meeting their nutritional needs through food alone, with the exception of vitamin D. And some kids who got supplements were absorbing zinc above the recommended upper limit. The study said chronic zinc overdoses may be tied to suppressed immune response and a decrease in the body's absorption of copper, which helps in the formation of red blood cells, among other functions.

Retrieved from:
http://online.wsj.com/article/SB100014240527487040932045752116680062403458.html

•Increased Breast Cancer Risk: Many women use multivitamins in the belief that these supplements will prevent chronic diseases such as cancer and cardiovascular disease. A recent prospective cohort study of 35,329 women observed a significant association between multivitamin use and an increased risk of breast cancer. Am J Clin Nutr (March 24, 2010).

•Men Overdosing, Increased Prostate Cancer Risk: Two of three men's multis failed to pass Consumer lab testing. One contained 258.8% of its folic acid, yielding 2,070 mcg per day. The RDA for folic acid is only 400 mcg per day and the upper tolerable level (UL) for folic acid is 1,000 mcg. Higher intake can make it difficult to detect severe vitamin B-12 deficiency. In addition, folic acid supplementation at 1,000 mcg per day has been associated with a more than doubling of the risk of prostate cancer.
Retrieved from:
http://www.consumerlab.com/news/Multivitamin_Multimineral_Test_Results/3_31_2009

It's not easy to simply change your lifestyle cold turkey (no pun intended) when you grow up in a society where vitamins are considered beneficial to health and meat is usually the main course of dinner. In restaurants, there are few selections for vegetarian dishes, and all of them seem to be pasta. So the answer doesn't necessarily have to be "go vegetarian". In reality, for the informed consumer, an easier, more convenient way to approach this dilemma is to redefine how you shop at your market and take a more informed approach to ordering food at a restaurant. Yes, some people say it requires a lifestyle change. Well, so does cutting off a woman's breast. If you make the effort to get the most out of the healthy foods you do consume, then indulging in that slice of triple chocolate something delectable once a year isn't really going to make or break your healthy lifestyle, and neither is taking a vitamin supplement**.

**The one exception for vegans is vitamin B-12 which used to be naturally occurring in soils. However, now that American soils are treated and diminished of the natural organisms that provide these important vitamins and minerals, some experts suggest the only necessary supplement is vitamin B-12.

Chapter 10: The Science

During a time span of about 4 weeks, a dear friend up-rooted her life and moved across the country within 3 days because her mother was diagnosed with cancer. Another friend's father was diagnosed with prostate cancer. Then another's husband was rushed to the ER suddenly for bypass surgery. The stark reality is, this is all around us, happening every day. It's almost as if there is this underground society, a world out there where people "in the know" throw around terms like "CSA" and "Braggs Liquid Aminos" as if those terms were average household conversation. In mainstream America, these are not yet common terms, yet the words "salad and breadsticks" makes just about every American think of one restaurant chain in particular. Is that good branding or is it contributing to the obesity epidemic?

Essentially, foods fall into just 3 categories, concentrated proteins and carbohydrates (read: meat and potatoes), high water content (read: fruits and vegetables) and fats (from oils to omega 3, 6, & 8 essential fatty acids). It's important to consider the basic guidelines about combining foods, not only because you might be on a health food kick, but because improper food combinations cause all kinds of problems from stomach aches, gas, reflux, constipation, and diarrhea to cancer cell multiplication; as benign as some of these symptoms seem, they are just that: symptoms of a larger problem.

Proper consumption of your healthy foods actually produces natural and healthy effects. The by-products of incomplete digestion from improper food combinations occurs in the small intestine and colon which turn into gases, then are transported through the intestinal walls into the bloodstream where they intoxicate the entire body.[16]

If an animal protein (chicken or pork for example) is consumed with a complex carbohydrate (read: Whole Grain) the different digestive juices in your body dilute each other's effectiveness, the protein is contaminated in the body (read: smells stinky) while the sugar ferments and produces gas. It's no wonder farting always seems to close the generation gap and make everyone laugh. Wow, that goes against everything you've ever learned right? Consider where you are learning that from, because a chain restaurant is banking on marketing a dinner to you while you're hungry. So what is the translation? If you haven't yet made the transition to plant-based, you can start slowly by allowing your meat to become a condiment instead of a main course; eat less of it, sliced on top of a salad or as a side dish with vegetables as your main course for optimal digestion.

The human body naturally balances its optimal weight when it is nourished properly. Diet fads and diet systems, along with food industry marketing techniques trick us into thinking their way is the right way, and that is precisely why someone who may have lost weight following the latest fad will tend to gain it back a short time later. It's not about diet, it's about re-educating yourself on how important nutrition is to overall well-being.

According to Pitchford (et, al.) there are two distinctly different types of digestion: an acid digestion for proteins (meat, fish, dairy) and an alkaline digestion for carbohydrates (sugars and starches). Proteins are mostly digested in the stomach, by an acidic gastric juice called hydrochloric acid. Another important ingredient of gastric juice is pepsin, which digests protein. A little known fact: if you are going to eat animal protein such as meat, you should definitely eat an acid fruit such as pineapple with your meat because the natural acids in the pineapple will help break down the meat so that it is easier to digest. Think about it...this is precisely why it works to marinate meat for a few hours before cooking it, for the acids to break down the meat. Carbohydrates, on the other hand, are not digested in the stomach, but are digested in the small intestine (mostly by pancreas secretions, which are alkaline). Further, fats digest differently - they leave the stomach largely unchanged but upon entering the small intestine cause the gall bladder to empty bile into the small intestine. Logically, if fat and carbs are both together in the intestine at the same time, they counter the effectiveness of one another.

Here is more interesting facts about food and digestion. Raw spinach and raw tomatoes are examples of foods which create a "good" alkaline in our bodies, but, it is important to know that these two vegetables actually change when they are cooked and produce something called "oxalic" acid which assists in digestion, but can also crystalize in the kidneys. When we have excess acid in our system, our bodies naturally produce cholesterol to balance the acidity. The body also produces fat to buffer the acid. Remember the same concept with the animal proteins and osteoporosis? Foods such as parsley and ginger help to keep the kidneys strong, while apple cider vinegar can help restore the acidic balance of the stomach. Interestingly, lemons, which we perceive to be highly acidic, digest and assimilate into alkaline within our bodies, which is good for us. The short of it is, when proper food combinations are ignored, your body cannot detoxify properly. But wait, there's more. Don't overcook your vegetables. Contrary to popular belief, you should not boil your vegetables in water on the stovetop. Instead, either eat the vegetables raw, or steam that broccoli for only about 3 minutes just to soften it up. It should have a dark, rich color and be slightly crunchy. If it's soft enough to melt in your mouth, then you cooked all the beneficial vitamins and minerals right out of it.

So what are the rules exactly, and how does the average person make sense out of the food combination rules? Consult the chart below to classify each food, and then follow the rules.

THE RULES OF FOOD COMBINING [16]

1. Sub acid fruits should be combined with acid fruits or sweet fruits. Sub acid fruits are apples, apricots, blueberries, cherries, kiwi, mangoes, peaches, pears and plums. Acid fruits are citrus, pineapple, raspberries and strawberries.

2. Do not combine acid fruits with sweet fruits. Sweet fruits include bananas, dates, figs, and raisins.

3. Melons should be eaten alone. The melon is the fastest digesting food. If you eat a meal and then have a few slices of watermelon for dessert, then the watermelon will immediately digest and leave the rest of the meal to rot in your stomach, causing bloating, fullness, and fatigue. Fruits, especially the melons contain simple carbohydrates (sugars) which monopolize all digestive functions so the other foods have to wait and ferment. All melon (watermelon, honeydew, cantaloupe, etc.) should be eaten alone, without any other foods. Think 2:00 pm snack in the middle of the day. You should not eat anything else after eating a melon for at least 2 hours.

4. Do not combine acids and carbohydrates. In other words, do not drink orange juice with toast or cereal. Non-starchy vegetables and ocean vegetables go with anything: proteins, oils and butter, grains, starchy vegetables, lemons and

126

limes. Think raw carrots with hummus, or collard greens sautéed in olive oil with salt and pepper.

5. Do not combine high protein (meat, fish, eggs, cheese) with starch (potato, pasta, bread, cereal) at the same meal. Proteins require acid for their digestion in the stomach, while carbohydrates require alkaline for digestion in the small intestine. Sugars inhibit the secretion of the hydrochloric acid in the stomach and combine with the free hydrochloric acid which interferes with the digestion of proteins. Conversely, if proteins are being digested in the stomach and there is more acid there for the sugar to combine with, then it will require much more alkaline secretion from the pancreas to neutralize the extra acid before it goes to work on the sugar. So what exactly does this mean? Avoid spaghetti and meatballs! For a healthier digestion, combine your pasta with eggplant and zucchini instead of meatballs.

6. All meat, milk, dairy, and eggs should be avoided (except mother's milk for infants). I know, this is a tough one. If you are healthy to begin with, you can start by cutting back; use a *minimal amount* of meat and dairy. If you have already been diagnosed or pre-diagnosed for disease...then obviously the recommendation is to cut out all meat and dairy.

7. Lettuce and celery are commonly thought to aid in the digestion of other foods. Ideally, you should eat a salad at the end of your meal rather than the beginning because the vegetables and presumably vinegar in the salad dressing will aid in the digestion of the starch and protein.

8. Be very careful and conscious of what children eat.
    A child's digestive system is very delicate, and
    many chronic diseases later in life including
    emotional and behavioral problems are the result of
    too much sugar, salt, fat, and processed food.

How to "Fix It"

- If you eat protein and starch during the same meal,
  for goodness sake, eat more vegetables!
- If you eat nuts, eat an acid fruit with them.
- If you still eat meat and dairy, eat it with an acid
  fruit such as pineapple.
- If you ate too much sugar, eat grapes.
- If you ate too much salt, eat watermelon.

How to Recognize It [16]

Following those rules can be tedious. It's a lot to remember.
Start with small substitutions, for example, like not adding
any melon to your fruit salad. Did you know the number one
clinical symptom of heart disease in men is erectile
dysfunction? Often times, people don't even recognize that
there is an underlying health problem because most of the
time they feel well. In fact, many times, people have been
living with some of these symptoms for such a long time,
that they don't even realize that these seemingly
insignificant signs are actually symptoms of a larger
problem.

Consider some of the following physical and emotional
signs and symptoms which typically suggest a weakness in
the liver from many years of eating foods that are unhealthy:

Physical Signs	**Emotional Signs**
allergies	anger
indigestion	frustration
stress, neck and back tension	resentment
fatigue	impatience
rigid, inflexible body	moodiness
impure blood, skin disorders	impulsiveness
finger/toenail problems	emotional attachments
muscular pain	poor judgment
slow to rise in the morning	mental rigidity
	negativity

Often times, these physical and emotional signs go unrecognized, or blamed on something else. It's kind of like that co-worker, the one who leads a life of imbalance, always angry, always moody. The excess, bad food that accumulates because of years of bad nutritional practices causes the imbalance which then in turn leads to unresolved sorrow. It's the first and easiest way to make a change for the better.

Exploring food combinations is one of the most magical and delicious simplicities of cooking. Chef Alain Chapel (1937-1990) is quoted saying "Cuisine is an act of love…You have to love either what you are going to eat, or the person you are cooking for." The seasons of the year make up an important component of well-being as well, because we are influenced by climate changes and the environmental elements. Also, the increasing availability of heirloom quality fruits and vegetables moves us toward achieving harmony with the food of different seasons.

Food has a therapeutic effect on the human body, and those who recognize this seem to discover that life is really about your experiences with others. If you generally feel well because of the foods you eat, you will be a happier person and have better experiences and interactions with others in your life. After all, those experiences *are* the essence of life...the *dance of all dances*.*

The "dance of all dances" is a phrase I first heard used by a professor at the University of Utah, Salt Lake City, UT. It was originally coined by L. Edna Rogers, as she refererred to the "art" of communication. I think that power is captured through human interaction when we're feeling well, and our overall wellness is directly related to the foods we eat.

The Question of Protein

One of the most frequently asked questions about the plant-based diet is "where do you get your protein?" Typically people believe that the more protein you get, the better. Why do people think that the human body needs so much protein? Well, about every 5 years, the Food and Nutrition Board of the Institute of Medicine (IOM) of the National Academy of Sciences in Washington, DC comes out with a report which determines the guidelines and health policies that suggest Americans should follow in order to minimize their risk for chronic diseases. The most current report available, as of the time of this writing, is actually from 2006, and it stipulates that the average adult should consume between 10-35% of their calories from protein.[30] The problem is, that same report five years ago indicated that the recommended daily allowance for protein was just 10% for average adults. That is a big difference. Why does it matter?

In order to determine how much protein average adults really need, scientists measure and compare the amount of nitrogen we consume with the amount of nitrogen we lose. Nitrogen is unique to protein, so what they actually do is measure the nitrogen as an index of protein intake. Protein turns over regularly, as the human body synthesizes new protein and gets rid of old protein, so yes, it must be replaced daily basis. But according to the science,[34, 35, 36, 37] the minimum daily requirement for the average adult to remain healthy is much less, a mere 5% – 6% of total calories. If you want to be really exact, researchers add to that number two statistical adjustments (called standard deviation) to assure that everyone else will still get the right amount, even though there are varying needs. So this measurement is more than adequate, theoretically and statistically speaking, for 98% of the population.

Incidentally, it turns out that people consume about 10% to 11% protein by eating plant-based foods.

By getting too much protein in your body, your other bodily systems have to work hard to remove the excess protein. This not only causes fatigue but it raises your cholesterol and effectively "turns on" the biological occurrences that lead to cancer cell division. Do you think this answers the question about why you may be feeling so tired at 3:00 in the afternoon...if you've eaten yogurt and a protein bar for lunch? Your body is busy working hard to eliminate the toxins of the meal you just consumed. Maybe you thought it was a healthy meal, except because there was so much animal-based protein (ie: milk, yogurt, eggs, meat) that is why your body feels tired, bloated, and irritable.

So now the question becomes, "how much protein do I usually consume?" It turns out that the average diet, in 95% of the U.S., has a range of protein intake from about 11% of total calories up to 22% of total calories per day. Why is the Food and Nutrition Board giving a number of 10-35% when the number should be less than 10%? Again, the answer comes down to politics.

Even when high ranking professionals stood up for the science behind the claim, the larger, more powerful institution won out and instead of providing accurate guidance backed by science, they decided that a range would suffice. Well now we're clearly learning that it doesn't suffice. If you want to be healthy, you have to educate yourself, otherwise you'll be off to seek medical treatment for your chronic disease. Maybe you've already started seeking treatment but nothing works. Maybe you didn't actually realize that some very important changes to what you eat on a daily basis could actually work.

Before you put down this book and resort to skepticism, I encourage you to try it for 10 days. Be honest with yourself though...eliminating cheese is not easy. Eliminating certain foods you've grown accustomed to eating over the past few decades is not easy. My husband's latest joke is that he would like to find a cheesesteak seed and plant it in our garden. He even envisions fresh Amoroso* rolls to go along with it. We're a Philly family through and through; thank goodness Amoroso has some whole grain options.

Amoroso Baking Company's hearth-baked bread rolls is a family-owned bakery located in Philadelphia, Pennsylvania. The bakery had it's humble beginnings in 1904, and over the last 100+ years (yep, thats right, and entire century) has grown into global distribution of it's breads.

Back to food combinations: so, you've eaten too much protein over the past few decades, you suffered from kidney stones or gall bladder problems; you've clearly caused damage to your internal organs that you didn't even realize was there. What can you do?

Foods that accelerate liver rejuvenation include chlorophyll-rich foods such as wheat grass and fresh vegetable juices as well as micro-algae spirulina and chlorella. These do not grow in the United States but can be found in health food stores. Fruit of course is a natural cleanse which can be used on a daily basis. Eat nothing but fruit in the morning, and then eat your whole grain cereal or toast about an hour later.

A practical way that I do this myself is to eat fresh fruit immediately when I get back from my morning run. Then, by the time I stretch and take a shower, I'm ready for the whole grain part of my breakfast: oatmeal and coffee.

Overcoming your arterial residues of fat and cholesterol (hypertension) obviously only occurs with a diet based on whole grains, fruits and vegetables combined with exercise. Therefore it is easy to conclude that if you have been diagnosed with any of the beginning diseases of the vascular system, it might be a good idea to incorporate the following foods into your diet. These foods for natural cleansing are suggested based on Eastern tradition:

- Mung Beans
- Peas
- Lentils
- Radish
- Garlic
- Celery
- Banana
- Seaweeds

Interestingly, there are vastly widespread ideas about foods which have certain cleansing properties. For example, it is believed that mung beans block a bodily mucus that builds up over time from eating a poor diet. It is also believed that large concentrations of vitamin b17 can be found in many beans, lentils, and in the seeds of apricots, apples, nectarines, cherries, peaches, pears, plums, and prunes. Vitamin b17 is widely used in countries other than the U.S. as a natural alternative for chemotherapy, sometimes called Laetrile Therapy. While the FDA (Food & Drug Administration) in the U.S. has used strict regulations (not law) to ban vitamin b17 over the years, it is found naturally occurring in certain foods. You're not going to find this at your local GNC.

It has, however, been clinically proven that certain foods do lend themselves to cancer prevention, especially cruciferous vegetables that contain "glucosinolates" and onions, and garlic which are rich sources of the potent anti-cancer bioflavonoid quercetin. [17] It is also widely believed that radishes have the ability to cleanse thick toxic mucus residues caused by eating animal products. Asparagus is a detoxifying and valuable diuretic for cleansing your system of the animal residue that feeds cancer cell growth. Other vegetables which have been recommended by the National Cancer Institute are: cabbage, turnip, kale, cauliflower, broccoli and brussels sprouts because they contain "dithiolthiones" a group of compounds which have anti-cancer, antioxidant properties. Cruciferous vegetables are rich in nutrients, including several carotenoids (beta-carotene, lutein, zeaxanthin); vitamins C, E, and K; foliate; and minerals. They also are a good fiber source.

"DON'T GET YOUR FUEL FROM THE SAME PLACE YOUR CAR DOES."

I think it's imperative to speak about dining out in America for a few moments. To borrow a bit of humor from the author of *In Defense of Food* (Michael Pollan, 2006) "Don't get your fuel from the same place your car does." I actually found this out the hard way when my husband got inducted into his college sports hall of fame.

We were on a 4 hour drive from our home to where he went to college when, after nearly 2 hours, we realized the only place to actually stop for food was a Sheetz. MTO right? If you know what that acronym stands for, then you might want to take a hard look at how many times you've purchased food from a gas station in the past year. How's that for altering your appetite? American gas stations make more money selling food than gasoline.

I was disappointed, on more than one occasion before I dove into the plant-based way of life, at the deshelved burger I received at a drive through, topped off by an angry clerk with a bad attitude. My take on that has always been that if I'm paying a premium for a prepared meal, at the very least I expect it to be consistent. This bias has evolved since my days of living on bagel sandwiches and coffee to my current state as a consumer of very few packaged and prepared foods. However I do place a extraordinary amount of value on restaurants that use fresh, local, sustainable ingredients. If I go out to dinner, you can bet my choice is not a chain restaurant. Listen up restaurateurs...we can taste the difference. Instead of including 40 choices on your menu, focus on a few key entrees made with local "farm to table" ingredients and hire a chef that knows how to transform those ingredients into a masterpiece, because exceptional food speaks for itself.

One of my friends, who never met my mother, recently said to me: "...we may not live in the fashion capital of the world, but we certainly do have access to fresh ingredients."

My mom, the queen of St. John, would have definitely appreciated that comment. Her spirit is ever-present in so many ways.

Part IV
The Cancer Mantra

CHAPTER II:
OUR IRREVERSIBLE MISTAKE

Why is hospital food so unhealthy, just like school cafeteria food? What prompted this chapter, and ultimately one of the driving forces behind my focus on researching plant-based nutrition is the story of the last 6 months of my mom's life. It is a story that is so painstakingly familiar to any family in which someone has been diagnosed with cancer, that as hard as it is, I have to share it. The bottom line is, I didn't know this, I wish it would have been shared with me, so now, I am sharing it with you.

Remember, information that is economically valued is what reaches the public. While it is widely known that vegetables, fruits, and whole grains, are believed to offer the best protection against various cancers, experts are still reluctant to acknowledge the primary importance of diet in the progression and reversal of cancer, and make nutrition a priority in the treatment plan of cancer patients. I obviously found this out first hand, the hard way.

My mother's team of physicians and oncologists, for both her breast cancer treatment as well as her bone-marrow transplant, never once provided us with a discussion about nutrition, except when we were told that she could not eat fresh fruits and vegetables during her chemo treatments because of the potential for the presence of bacteria which could be harmful to her compromised immune system. Cancer patients will be familiar with the term "neutropenia" which means an abnormally low count of neutrophils or white blood cells that help your immune system fight off infections, particularly of bacteria and fungi. The idea is that these bacteria are present in fresh foods, so the physicians recommend eating only packaged foods. Wow. How about that for contradictory information. And these are some of the top cancer treatment programs in the country.

Intuitively, my mom seemed to know there was something wrong with this picture, as I can vividly recall her questioning why the hospital fed her chocolate pudding instead of a banana. I realize I can't look back, but sometimes this very question of hospital food versus fresh food just haunts every facet of my well-being. Overcoming disease is not only about strength and will to live, my mom had those...as do so many cancer patients that I have known personally. I remember these conversations with her as if they happened yesterday. Of course I do, nearly every discussion centered around food in my family; what is amazing to me is that she almost had a sixth sense, she knew that good food made her feel better. Even though at times she was taking up to 20 pills a day, she recognized that the pills were making her feel worse and the food was making her feel better. The difference now is very personal for me.

The first series of events in 2001 happened very fast. My mom was 51 years old at the time; first came a lump, then a diagnosis, then surgery a few weeks after that. We trusted a team of physicians at one of the most prominent breast cancer facilities in our nation. They told us one of the long-term side effects of chemo was the potential for additional cancers, but, the prognosis for a quick surgery and treatment plan would essentially save her life in the short term. What they didn't emphasize was that cancer is identified in three stages: initiation, promotion, and progression.

The promotion stage may take years from the time the initiated mutated cell first replicates itself until the time it grows into a troublesome tissue mass, and, one of the most important features of promotion is its reversibility.

140

Looking back now, I know the surgery didn't need to happen immediately, but lack of knowledge encourages fear, and as a family, we feared the worst: losing her.

LACK OF KNOWLEDGE ENCOURAGES FEAR.

She followed the professional course of treatment and the advice of the physicians, had the mastectomy and underwent chemotherapy. Treatments, follow-up visits, hair loss, pills, and side effects, yet willpower prevailed. She was a true survivor. From 2002 to about 2006, if you didn't know her personally, you never would have known my mom was a cancer survivor.

Fast forward five years, my mom was feeling like she had the flu for about 3 weeks. After several more weeks of tests and diagnostic procedures, her health declining rapidly, our family internist discovered something significant. Multiple blood transfusions in our local hospital followed, and she was rushed, again, to one of the premier cancer facilities on the east coast where they determined the diagnosis was Acute Myeloid Leukemia, a blood cancer that developed because of the chemo treatments from her breast cancer, years prior. I was seven months pregnant when this happened; it was New Year's Eve, 2006. I sat with her in the hospital, believing she would recuperate in time for the birth of my first baby...her first grandchild...due in 3 months. First, more chemo. My father and I took turns driving her more than an hour and a half each way to the hospital on a daily basis for treatments and appointments. Then came their recommendation: A bone-marrow transplant. She was placed on the waiting list while the chemo treatments resumed. It seemed this was the best course of action under the circumstances, because really, what other choice did we have? What other choice do all cancer patients have?

WHAT OTHER CHOICE

DO CANCER PATIENTS HAVE?

This is the part where you learn from my family's painful and irreversible mistake. Exchange your fears for the hope that arises when you have reliable knowledge, and I encourage you to have an honest and productive discussion with your team of physicians about real solutions instead of just accepting the bias and false consensus of western medicine. This is especially true for men. Women, by nature, tend to be much more conversational about emotionally charged discussions while men become disengaged or simply keep their fears hidden. There is power and strength in your soul gentlemen, and it is the source of life and passion; stop neglecting it.

The once thought of as "alternative" options to chemotherapy, radiation, and surgery are now much more widely accepted, and with good reason. Contrary to mainstream belief, most cancer patients really are afforded enough time to thoroughly research their options.* Major scientific research experiments have been conducted over the past decade that indicate that intake of fruits, vegetables (and consequently on the negative side of the equation, animal protein) actually controls the promotion of cancers initiated by various other causes, and further, returning the body to optimal levels of consumption of certain nutrients can halt or even reverse progression. This relationship between diet and cancer was not discussed with us during my mom's treatment, not even once. Hmm. So, one of the leading causes of death in America is not really cancer, it is ignorance about nutrition?

As different perspectives guide the questions we ask, they also to some extent dictate the answers that we actually find.

During the course of my research for this book, I interviewed yet another dear friend and breast-cancer survivor. I pointedly asked her whether discussions about nutrition was a fundamental part of her treatment plan. Not only was nutrition not part of her treatment either, it confirmed my assumptions that even the highest educated medical practitioners are confused about the relationship between diet and disease, and that most treatment plans lack consideration of something so basic as proper nutrition as actually being a factor in prevention and healing. Another interviewee who prefers to remain anonymous did mention that while nutrition wasn't specifically discussed as part of her medical plan, she felt that may be due to the fact that her disease was diagnosed in the very early stages; she felt that perhaps other cancer patients might expect to have nutrition discussed in the later stages of diagnosis. I don't know about you, but I would like to see it discussed sooner than later.

---

*For more information on the topic of alternative treatment, please see The Moss Reports, under the Additional Resources section on page 225.

The Nutrition Ideology

Why does the Standard American Diet make us sick? The Center for Disease Control and Prevention has kept a database over the last decade which has progressively shown steady up-ticks in obesity and further forcasts that 32 million more Americans will be obese by the year 2030. People need to recognize that nutrition is not an ideology; it is not simply meal planning, but rather a word indicative of the integrated effects of countless dietary and lifestyle factors, all acting together in harmony. Even the biochemical and physiological effects of stress illustrate yet another dynamic linked to nutrition which is part of overall wellness. Stress has become so interwoven into everyday suffering that we as a society have come to accept as normal. We need to begin by rediscovering the importance of the mind-body connection.

Consequently, someone else I know founded a breast cancer rehabilitation clinic which focuses on the unique rehabilitative needs of mastectomy patients. As a result of our discussions, the program is now focusing on training its practitioners about the importance of plant-based nutrition.

Sometimes I think the entire cancer industry is counter-intuitive, or put another way, what we do instinctively achieves the opposite of the desired result. Why do we as a society pour millions of dollars into cancer research? I enthusiastically organized my own cancer fundraising event in 2008, and together with other family members raised thousands of dollars which was donated to cancer research. It doesn't seem to make a lot of sense. These large conglomerates seem to be looking for answers in the wrong places. The research focuses on finding a drug, a simple cure, because it's the way to make money. So much money that an entire industry has formed around a disease that employs as many people as lives that it takes.

Another important fact that we did not hear about directly from our team of physicians was that cancer initiators, in other words, the things we believe cause cancer, have been overemphasized so much that we as a society pretend that we don't really know the exact causes cancer. This is a myth. We know that cancer-promoting substances, such as nutrient imbalances, have a greater influence on cancer occurrence than the environmental chemicals, or carcinogens which cause the cancer in the first place.

What exactly does that mean? Well, you can either change your diet or die of toxicity to all other systems of your body from chemotherapy. It's not cancer that kills people, it is the poison to all of the other healthy bodily systems that slowly degenerates the entire body until the body just can't take anymore. Why do people choose to poison themselves? Because they don't understand the disease. Why do well meaning medical practitioners allow people to do this to themselves? Ask your practitioner what he would do if he were in your shoes, and then listen carefully to how he phrases the answer to that question.

CHAPTER 12: THE ART OF HEALING

Life balance can be very complex. It equates to different things for different people, and is highly dependent upon your situation, your age, and your life stage. It is my view that whatever the circumstances of your life may be, understanding how to achieve balance is truly the purest form of harmony and wellness within you. Choosing the right foods can help us achieve balance in other dimensions of our life, and this balance brings inner contentment, a sense of calm, peace, and happiness.

Sometimes peace simply comes from silence. Obviously if you're a parent you know this. We're so busy with technology, our smartphones nestled comfortably by our bedside, that it's a miracle we even get a full, restful night sleep. We rarely take time out of our busy schedule to take a personal inventory of the different factors that actually contribute to our happiness, and how those factors stack up to what is most important in our lives. We need that brief moment of silence to reflect, heal, and nourish our soul on a daily basis.

There is an old cliche…Life is not measured by the number of breaths we take, but by the moments that take our breath away. Those are powerful words, especially when unexpected cataclysmic events suddenly arise that remind us how precious life can be.

I would like to share with you a partial list of the side effects (read: quality of life issues) of the leading chemotherapy treatments which I observed, first hand:

Side Effects of my mother's Chemotherapy treatments:

1. bleeding
2. bruising
3. fatigue
4. neutropenia
5. diarrhea
6. vomiting
7. mouth sores
8. bed sores
9. increased risk of infection
10. advice to specifically "not" eat certain whole foods because of the increased risk of infection due to a comprimised immune system

What I learned once I actually had the time to reflect on my mother's course of treatments is that today, much more than 10 or even 5 years ago, it is widely known that cancer patients are not dying of cancer, they are dying of toxicity to so many other parts of the body. If there is one fact that you take away from reading this book, I hope it is this one:

CANCER PATIENTS ARE NOT

DYING OF CANCER,

THEY ARE DYING OF TOXICITY TO

SO MANY OTHER PARTS OF THE BODY.

The fact is, and I've mentioned this already, the cancer industry has become so lucrative that it actually employs more people than it helps. Did you know that oncologists are able to buy chemotherapy drugs and administer them in their own clinics as an alternative to sending patients to the hospital to receive treatment?

It is estimated, according to a lecture by Pamela A. Popper, N.D., Ph.D., that 2/3 of the oncologist's income is from the resale of chemotherapy drugs. In other words, referring patients to alternative therapy is not in their best interest because it obviously reduces their income.

So how does treatment become impartial and objective for the patient? It's easy to say that people should get second, third, and fourth opinions about treatment, but that is not easy to do that when you are right smack in the middle of it.

Speak to someone who has been recently diagnosed, and you'll find that a team of medical experts urging the patient to begin treatment immediately. I have a one word answer for why that works: Fear.

Further down the road, when it gets to the point where a patient is lying helpless in the intensive care unit with a trache tube down her throat, having eaten nothing but processed chocolate pudding for nearly 5 months, it's not easy for the decision makers in the family to think rationally. Allow me to reiterate...these intense side effects my mom experienced were not caused by the cancer itself, *they were caused by the chemotherapy*. But the question still remains... if you or a loved one is stricken with disease... what questions do you ask?

Oh dear God, the trache. I can't even begin to describe how painful it was to watch, so instead of describing that pain, I'll tell you what I did. I was 9 months pregnant with my son, just a few weeks away from giving birth, and my daughter was about to turn 1. I decided that I wanted to get my daughter's ears pierced, figuring she wouldn't be scared since she was barely a year old. My mom, you see, was one of those traditional people who thought that if God wanted the extra hole in your ear then he would have put it there.

She lived all 57 years of her life without having her ears pierced. I got mine pierced when I was 12. Trache tube aside, the non-verbal laughter that my mom and I shared that day, the day I walked into her hospital room, 9 months pregnant, with a 1-year old daughter with bling on her ears, was enough to keep her holding on just a bit longer. My mom couldn't speak, but I could read her like a book. It was almost like she was saying "I don't really care about the ears, I am confident in your ability to make your own decisions about parenting your children." I will never forget that day. It was the last day I saw her. My son was born shortly thereafter, and for nearly 2 weeks, I didn't go to the hospital for a visit. With a newborn and a 14 month old, I was a little busy. One sunny afternoon, my dad called and said that my mom wanted to speak to me. In a raspy voice (the trache had just been removed) she told me that I was "a good mommy" and that she loved me. All I could do was cry and tell her that I wanted her to come home. That was the last time I spoke to her.

I learned of a gentleman by the name of Ralph Moss, who was the assistant director of public affairs at Memorial Sloan-Kettering Cancer Center in New York from 1974-1977. He has independently evaluated the claims of conventional and non-conventional cancer treatments with research collected over the past 30 years. I wish someone had told me this five years ago, because it certainly would have been a good place to begin. Remember, I was 7 months pregnant when my mom was first diagnosed with AML. I had some other things on my mind, at the time, clearly not realizing what would soon be the series of events that would forever change my life.

Loosing a parent is not easy for anyone at any age. It's compounded a bit when you loose your mom and her namesake is only 2 weeks old, but the one legacy she left

150

with me was her resolve. She taught me that if you want to make a difference in your own life, you have to start with yourself. This is such an important lesson and involves all four of the fundamental wellness categories: nutrition, exercise, sleep, and mental balance.

IF YOU WANT TO MAKE A DIFFERENCE

IN YOUR OWN LIFE,

YOU HAVE TO START WITH YOURSELF.

Whether you consider meditation, religion, exercise, or simply sitting on the beach, taking a few moments to reflect can provide much needed stress therapy for the many different parts of your life that bring about stress. People who are busy seem to forget this important element.

It is so important to recognize that any type of stress contributes to significantly to disease, whatever that disease may be, so understanding how to properly manage yourself and your own emotional wellbeing first is just the beginning of a healthier, happier, you. Each case of disease is unique, although modern medical practice seems to classify so many of them together. Many times, principles are applied across the board, without regard to whether a particular course of treatment is really best suited to a person's medical condition. Anyone who has made an appointment to see a doctor, only to sit in the waiting room for an eternity and then only to have received a few minutes of their time knows that it would be impossible to begin anywhere but with yourself first. Symptoms vary widely, so it is essential to heal by observation, listening on many different levels (non-verbal) and exercising care and patience while at the same time, applying the practices the professionals were trained in. In some circles, and in Eastern traditions, this is called Alternative, Natropath, or Holistic medicine. I cannot stress

151

the importance of seeking out a physician or team of medical practitioners who practice natropathic and preventative care.

It's about preventative care. Preventative. PREVENTATIVE.

Today, we are merely a statistic, rushed in, seen often times by a practitioner who is not even the doctor, and rushed out with a prescription in hand, only to find so many side effects that it's a wonder if that prescription was really right for us anyway. Another lesson I learned from my mother, is that intuition plays a vital role in healing, so it is even more important to find that health care provider who really cares to listen. Perhaps if more Americans took an active role in their own well being instead of a "pill for every ill" they would notice that what we eat directly relates to the big picture of our overall wellness. It's not easy to do, and when you think about it, most people don't really care that much until it touches them personally. Some people think it's extreme that I am highly particular about the foods my children consume or that I am over the top about educating my children on proper nutrition. I think it's extreme that the hospital bill for one patient can cost millions of dollars while we sat helplessly and watched her die because they fed her nothing but pudding for 5 months.

We can do something about this, but it has to start with each individual. Perhaps we wouldn't have a healthcare crisis in the United States if 30% of our population wasn't obese. Why is our hard-earned money going to offset the cost of expensive surgeries and treatments for people who make the wrong choices?

I had a recent encounter with an uninspiring co-worker and wondered: what creates such imbalance? Each day in our daily professional lives, we strive to treat employees fairly, we recognize and respect the diversity of our workforce and the individualism of each person while maintaining a dominant market position and continued profitable growth. We are committed to filling each position with the most capable person available. Individual initiative, willingness and the ability to take responsibility, performance, and maintaining a strong communication link between all levels of the organization are criteria for success. But why is it that some people are so good at taking personal responsibility, have a charismatic, shining outlook on life, while others are dull and boring? Why do some people make the wrong choices when so man of us want so badly to make the right choices?

I am not an educator by trade, but what I've found is that my passion for both food and wellness has evolved throughout my life into educating people, families, and especially children about why eating whole foods is so important to every aspect of their well being. The fact is, happy, charismatic people breed happiness. I believe the benefit of both proper nutrition and exercise in children extends so much further than what we have come to imagine. Our children grow up to be those people in the workplace that either contribute or not. How do we teach our children to eat healthy and exercise? We model the behaviors. It is in the context of these interactions, with food, with loved ones, with the arts, and with sports that actually creates meaning for children, building their self image, coloring their experiences with positive emotions and giving them something to look forward to in life.

In my family, we're addicted to sports, but we must balance that with the other fundamental building blocks of well-being, because if we succomb to the "I don't have time to make dinner" syndrome, then all bets are off. Unless we impress proper habits in children from the very beginning, these actions and behaviors (toward food, sports, or respect

153

for themselves and others) assimilate and then disappear only to preserve such pragmatism in memory. Essentially, the overlap in these interconnections is what forms the basis of character and values which extend the reach of discipline, dedication, ingenuity, perseverance, and patience into the academic world, the community, and into adulthood, shaping their future, yet revolving around the complexities of interpretation from the primary years.

As parents, we must understand the importance of interpretation and instill positive values of respect and teamwork in our children. How do we do that? Can you give me an example besides modeling behavior about food?

What about stepping back and allowing a coach to do his job without adding your two cents as a spectator? If you think you know more about coaching your son or daughter's team than the coach does then why don't you apply for the job? Do your credentials mirror that of the coach? Do you even know what the coaches credentials are? Did you graduate from college while participating in a collegiate level sports training program, or further, a professional athletic program and carry a high grade point average at the same time? If you didn't, then you should stick to your day job and remain a spectator. The world is full of choices, and a coach has made that career choice. You could have made that choice too. Remember, parents, that individuals are socialized into the world by direct experience and sociobiological (or genetic) factors. So although it appears there is a link between attitude and behavior, what is it that you believe drives perception? The answer is how you model behavior to your children. How long must we wallow in a confused and angry sea of observation with no prospect of navigating a more peaceful and serene context? Get with the program, parents. It is you; you are ultimately responsible for the way your children act. If you shout profanities at the individuals who commit their time and effort to the betterment of your children, what message does that send to your children? If you don't buy fresh fruit and vegetables and you buy packages of processed food, what message does that send to your children?

I'm getting back to the point. The discipline of any sport can be cathartic, rejuvenative, almost harmonizing in the utilitarian system of unregulated egoistic capitalism that we live in today. What we parents need to remember is that the values learned through the involvement with sport create the basis not only for endurance, collaboration, and synergy on the field, but for altruism, fortitude, and tenacity in society. Choices about food go right along with choices about self control. If we all use those endorphins to give a little more without expectation, to encourage balance instead of adversarialism, I think there would be more children who grow up as vibrant, sophisticated, ethical professionals instead of drab, lifeless haters.

Reach into your Soul

to find your own
Moment of Silence

Today, more than ever before, I hear people say they need to "get to the gym". We all know that no matter where you choose to exercise, be it a fitness facility or outdoors, the benefits of regular exercise will not only benefit you but also your family. You will feel better and that directly translates to the ability to lessen the amount of stress from other areas of your life because you can manage your feelings. In terms of modeling behavior for overall wellness, when the parents exercise and eat right, children do the same. When parents practice excess, so do their children.

If you simply begin with a moment, 5 minutes a day of pure, unadulturated silence, it can work wonders for your overall well being.

Here are five ways you can fit that moment into your busy day:

1. Take 5 minutes after you exercise to stretch and elongate your muscles. While you stretch, inhale deeply and close your eyes. Clear your mind of all thoughts. Exhale and let go of everything.

2. Take 5 minutes while you're eating your morning breakfast or drinking your coffee. Instead of grabbing something on the way out the door, set your alarm 10 minutes earlier, so you have those few extra moments in the morning. Put down the newspaper, or sit down when you would instead be rushing to your car. Take a deep breath. Clear your mind. Then regroup and write down what you have to accomplish that day. Sometimes people underestimate the power of a to-do list that is actually written down.

3. Take a break at work. If you're simply too busy and you eat lunch at your desk, you most definitely need to take a 10 minute break. Go outside, even if it's raining, and take a short walk. Clear your mind. Take a deep breath. The rain will wash away anything if you let it.

4. If you find yourself yelling at your children, take a time out for yourself instead. Let them make a mess. Let them run around the house and be loud. Let them be children. Make sure they are safe, and then go in a room by yourself and close the door for 5 minutes. Take a deep breath. Let go of the notion of perfection. When I was growing up, my mother had a picture frame with the words: A clean house is the sign

of a life misspent. I didn't realize what that meant until I became a mother myself. Unfortunately, (or fortunately depending upon how you look at it) it was too late to thank her, but it was not to late to realize what it meant. It took me just a moment of silence to realize my 4-year old batman isn't for sale anymore.

5. Finally, if you can't find time during your busy day, take those 5 minutes when you lay down at night to sleep. Put your phone in another room. Clear your mind. Stop going over and over your day in your head, and stop thinking about what you have to do tomorrow. Instead, clear your mind. Imagine yourself in a place that you find comfort, whether it's relaxing on your couch or your favorite childhood place to be alone with your thoughts. Go back to that place in your mind, the place where you felt safe.

In an economy where more people are losing jobs than gaining them, retirement plans are on a downward spiral, and people are struggling to stay ahead of their own personal finances, giving serious consideration to how fruits and vegetables fit into your life isn't necessarily on the top of the list. Yet it is the nurturing of this very garden where the answer lies.

If you really take a moment to reach inside your soul, you will probably find that you are the only one who controls the type of life you lead.

It takes a lot of work to clean vegetables and fruits. If you're the kind of person who gives your apple a rinse under the kitchen sink, it's not enough. You need to scrub it with a vegetable brush and soap, until you can feel the sliminess dissappear and the skin get sticky.

I suppose 40 years ago people didn't obsess over whether the skin of the apple felt sticky or slimy, but 40 years ago

American soil wasn't contaminated with pesticides like it is today.

Wellness is a choice; I challenge you to start with that small block of time, 5 minutes each day to clear your head, couple that with The Plant Pledge (page 68) and begin your journey toward emotional and personal fulfillment. If you surround yourself with people who see the glass half empty, you too are conditioned to see the glass half empty. Remember, control how you speak to yourself in your own mind, otherwise it will control you.

Plant your own garden, watch how it fosters meaningful relationships and sustains your soul. Within each of us lies the power to change our circumstances, whatever they may be. Don't ever give sanction to sarcasm, devaluation, and negativity about your decision to change your eating habits and be well. Remember, it's your choice.

Part VI

Motivation:

Celebrate the Delectable Plant

CHAPTER 14:
WHAT TO EXPECT WHEN YOU GO PLANT

When I first began eating a plant-based diet, I decided to go to the bookstore to find a good vegan cookbook. Seems logical enough. Definitely not one of my best ideas. Going to the bookstore blindly in search of such a broad topic without an actual recommendation of an author/chef is like searching google with a phrase like "best restaurant in NYC." Boolean operators aside, I spent time flipping through the vegan cookbooks and eventually picked a few out strictly because the photos of the food looked good. Nice strategy right. I might as well browse Pinterest. I didn't know what "liquid smoke" was or where to find nutritional yeast, and I wasn't really sure what was in the "meatless" burger. Okay, well, not everyone has formal chef training at a culinary school in France, so in order to make sense of how to begin preparing food this way, I needed to better understand the essence of the more limited ingredients.

Having spent the better part of my childhood learning the fundamentals of cooking, baking, and entertaining from my mother proved to be a good foundation for taking over when it was time. The year she died, I stepped in to take over as hostess for the holiday that had been my moms for the past 35 odd years…Christmas Eve. Every year, my sister and I helped her prepare a homemade meal; what we didn't realize was that some of the ingredients we were using were really dangerous. Manicotti crepes from scratch, filled with a spinach and ricotta mixture, and served with a side of veal scallopini. That was the main course, and it was served along side an array of homemade appetizers including crab dip, gorgonzola crustini, anti-pasta, shrimp cocktail and a fancy salad. Sounds good right?

Both of my parents understood flavor affinities, and their use of herbs and spices, along with the syntax of perfect combinations really brought the occasion together. I think that is part of what made those moments so meaningful to me. The combination of the togetherness of family and the smells of the season all factor in to making an occasion memorable; that is ultimately the recipe for a magical celebration. So how exactly do you move your entire family from the foods you ate at those celebrations over the past few decades to healthier options? I'll be upfront with you right here and now…it is not an easy task.

When it was my turn to take over that Christmas Eve dinner (not by choice obviously) the first year was the hardest; tears streamed down with every ingredient, every cookie in the oven, and every glass on the table. I served up all of our traditions at that meal. Probably because my mom's essence was still with me, even though she wasn't there. The following year, my father decided that it was time to change the menu. Still not plant-based, I served meat as the main course: beef wellington with a duxelles filling. No big deal…only a formal sit-down Christmas Eve dinner for 30. Remember, I'm not a chef, just a person who appreciates good food. *You can imagine my initial skepticism about vegans.*

Let's face it, not only does it take a lot of work to clean vegetables, it takes a lot of work to be a vegan, much more than being a vegetarian. But what I ultimately discovered is that my mother's essence is present in every meal I prepare, whether it was her recipe or one I came up with myself. I realized that I could re-create the flavor combinations that the family grew accustomed to celebrating, and then pair healthier ingredients together with her as my inspiration.

There is a term gaining more popularity of late called a "flexitarian" — a carnivore who eats meat once or twice a week. In the very beginning of my research, as we considered moving from a meat-based diet to a plant-based diet, we gave this a try. However, once I dove in further, I realized how important it was to cut back significantly on the animal products. This is also where I learned about the term "junk" vegan. I mentioned this before in the food combination chapter, but what exactly does junk vegan mean? Well, suppose you decide to eat "vegan" because it seems healthy, so you eliminate the meat and dairy from your diet, but then you go to a restaurant and order french fries, because gosh, french fries fit into the category of a vegetable so they must be healthy, right? Okay, a french fry might be vegan, but it's not a health food, doesn't matter how you slice it. You sort of have to take veganism in stride. Remember, I'm not a fan of those vegan recipes that attempt to re-create the look and feel of the standard American foods. Just because your meatless balls look like meatballs and you serve them alongside pasta with tomato sauce and cashews that are crushed up to look like Parmigiano-Reggiano, it doesn't mean that meal is health food. Are you still with me?

So the moral of the story is, if you currently still eat meat, lets begin your journey down the path to wellness by eating a whole-foods, plant based diet instead of a "vegan" diet. If your goal is to not eat animals, then being a vegan makes sense, but in terms of health and wellness, a meatless ball is still a meatless ball.

It took me about ten months of trying out recipes for a vegan-burger (I mean a plant-based burger) before I actually found one that I liked; there are so many variations, from mushrooms to chickpeas to blackbeans.

163

What you need to know is this: just like learning to cook a gourmet meal from scratch requires years of practice, so does learning to cook a gourmet *vegan* meal.

My family and friends can attest to my customary bite when it comes to the chefs we sometimes see on television…you know the ones who simply bought a can of something off a grocery store shelf, added it to a bowl, mixed it with a few other store bought ingredients, and called it cooking.

For a brief moment, I thought about taking Aunt Mary's advice and creating a show of my own. Okay, that moment is over. I wouldn't last a hot red second next to Bobby Flay; but what I'm trying to say here is that there are plenty of mothers out there who truly understand how difficult it is to prepare meals day in and day out for your family.

We do the grocery shopping, clean the produce when we get home, peal and chop the ingredients, and then scour Pinterest for some ideas on how to make it into something that we hope is as decadent as the love that went into the preparation. It's not like the ingredients are just sitting there in a bowl already cleaned and chopped to the right consistency waiting for us to add them to the pan, in a nice clean kitchen I might add.

Many of us can look at a recipe and determine its potential simply by reading the list of ingredients. The good news is, if you already have the foundation, then the transition to eating more plant-based foods will be even easier. I never needed a recipe book to whip up dinner because I already had the foundation to make up my own recipes based on whatever happened to be in my fridge at any given moment. This is how you transform the food your family eats into something special, by paying special attention to the ingredients, respecting the farmer who grew those ingredients, and keeping sustainability in mind. I read an article recently by Anne-Marie Slaughter, titled *Why Women Still Can't Have it All*. She made the point that women **can** still have it all, just not *all at the same time*. I think that statement speaks to all women, no matter where you're at in your life. Whether you're still looking for jeans that make your butt look good or whether you need ideas about where to put your elf on the shelf, the reality of it is, we're ultimately all looking for the same thing.

Everything changes when you move to a plant-based diet. So now you know what you can expect, as far as cooking goes; over the short term, you will have to literally re-learn how to cook and bake. Baking is actually easier than cooking because most of the time, baking requires you to follow a recipe very precisely. One of the nice things about vegan baking is you can easily substitute things like applesauce for oil or bananas for eggs. This is not so in cooking, there is just no substitute for bacon.

There are recipe books, blogs and people out there who claim to "eat clean" or "pure" but then they publish recipes that contain ingredients like eggs and milk. Are these folks serious? Lets get this out of the way right here and now: Eating clean means eating fruits, vegetables, legumes, nuts, and whole grains. That's it. Period. End of story. Eggs are not pure. Chicken is not clean, and a genetically modified cracker is not whole. You ate a whole apple? That's great, and did you know that a slice of that same apple is still a whole food too? Oh, and a sprinkle of cinnamon on top, you know, the kind that comes from the bark of the Cinnamomum tree, is better than a sprinkle of sugar. Gosh there goes the cynicism again; all you really need to do is focus on recipes that celebrate the delectable plant.

FOCUS ON RECIPES THAT CELEBRATE THE DELECTABLE PLANT.

There is really so much more to eat than salad, with just a little guidance, you'll discover how elegant and distinctive plant-based recipes will taste. Contrary to popular belief, eating plant-based food does not mean that you live solely on twigs and berries. Think of it in terms of the experience; instead of lamenting about not being able to eat your favorite cheese that you've been eating every day of your life for the past 25 years, consider all of the compelling reasons while you'll never look back; you'll never waiver, and you'll become truly motivated to uproot your entire refrigerator and move toward plant-based foods.

Remember, a good cook doesn't necessarily follow a recipe, she evaluates the ingredients and then decides what to make. By learning about your local CSA (Community Supported Agriculture) you'll expose yourself to the types of ingredients that are local and in season in whatever part of the country you live in. Many CSAs even provide recipes to go along with the foods they are growing. I love my CSA, it reminds me of Christmas when I was a child...you never know what you're going to get, so when you open that box each week, you are surprised by all the gorgeous produce. You're inspired to seek out new and interesting recipes, and you have those fresh, healthy ingredients right at your fingertip.

There is something very comforting about ritual. Especially if you've been cooking and eating the same way for most of your adult life. But everything changes in an instant when the foreseeability of disease enters the equation.

Fear takes over. Or maybe it doesn't, and then someone you care deeply about dies suddenly of a heart attack or is stricken by cancer. It's time to break the cycle. It's time to take control of the things you do have control over...like what you feed your family. An apple costs less than a breakfast bar and will keep you full much longer. Vegetables aren't sexy, but if it's vanity that you care about, then you might just be tempted by how sexy you'll look after a few weeks of eating those vegetables versus a few weeks of cheeseburgers. Choosing the right types of foods will help you achieve balance in so many other areas of your life, isn't that what ritual is really about?

Chapter 15: The Power of Yes!

Now that you've got an essential foundation about why dairy is the devil, and overall wellness is deeply rooted in proper nutrition, you're ready to give it a try. Whether you're completely convinced and ready to dive in head first or whether you're still skeptical and want to try out a few small changes, I want to help you get there. I want to help you get your family there. I understand how difficult it is to make these changes, especially when you've been eating a certain way for the past decade or more.

This next chapter focus' on how and where to actually begin your journey, and then the charts and recipes at the back of the book will provide you with some guidance to get started on the road to better health and well being.

So here we are, ready to begin. You've made the decision to eat clean, as soon as you're done reading this book you're gong to toss all the bad items out of your fridge, and stock it with new foods that you may have never heard of before, and what can you actually expect to happen? For starters, you'll actually being saving some money on food. I can feed a family of 4 on about $185 a week. That is 28 breakfasts, 28 lunches, and 28 dinners for $185. For the math majors, that is $2.20 per person, per meal. If you plant a garden, bonus, you just cut your grocery bill even more.

One of the first most noticeable agenda items is the brief period of adjustment your body needs to adapt to your new way of eating. When you make any sudden change in the foods you eat, it's always a shock to the system. Give yourself some time, anywhere from a few days to a few weeks because everyone is different. In fact, you may actually need to ease into it instead.

Some people believe that healthier foods cause more flatulence. This is an old wives tale. There are theories out there that eating more fiber is a shock to the system or that beans and cruciferous vegetables like broccoli or cabbage cause gassiness. In reality, it isn't the food that causes the gas, it's the reaction of the enzymes that are produced with the gastric juices in your stomach and intestines. Remember, there are guidelines for the combination of certain foods which have a direct impact on digestion, refer back to Chapter 10, The Science.

Because of the regenerative qualities of chlorophyll rich foods, plants help to discharge the body of animal toxins. Whole foods, along with their color, aroma, and healing properties will clean, build, and renew your body. That is reason enough to become more intimate with your produce! It is important to note, however that a common problem which results in digestive weakness is the gross overuse of fruits and their juices. Fruit is cleansing by nature, so it should be consumed in smaller amounts than vegetables. Additionally, fruit is naturally sweet, stop adding sweetener! Chemical additives actually speed deterioration of organ systems within your body, once your body can no longer tolerate the excess, it begins to malfunction and causes a deficiency of vitamins and minerals. Inflammation. Auto-immune dysfunction. Irritable bowel syndrome. Migraines. Arthritis. Allergies to certain foods. Sometimes even symptoms that were barely noticeable before begin to clear up with a plant-based diet. You never realized that cheese was the culprit, or that grazing on just a few crackers for a mid-day snack was really tricking your body into being hungrier.

Move those apprehensions to the side and get ready to feel better than ever before.

5 STEPS GET YOU STARTED:

STEP 1:   Drop your fear at the end of this chapter.

You can't move forward if you're still not convinced that meat and dairy cause cancer and heart disease. For those of you who need additional resources, check out the Resources and References sections at the back of the book to find additional information.

STEP 2: Clean out your fridge and your pantry.

Remember the simple rule, if it's not in your house, you can't eat it. Perhaps even more importantly, **if you don't buy it, your children can't eat it!** Don't go to the grocery store with your children. If proper nutrition is going to be a priority for your family, then schedule a time to go grocery shopping when you can do it alone, without your children. Sometimes as parents, we forget how hard it is to actually **focus** when children are around us. You'll be amazed at the peace and serenity you can have for an hour in the grocery store without the children there to rush you.

What should you keep in your fridge and pantry? The list of starter recommendations follows this chapter.

STEP 3: Make your commitment public.

That's right, announce it on Facebook, or twitter, or whatever social network you use. Tell your friends and your family that you have decided to change your life. It's a big

171

deal, and you will feel better about your decision to make some changes if there are people out there to support you along the way. Instead of Facebook friends poking fun at your choice of ordering a vegetable wrap at the baseball game when they order a cheesesteak and fries, they will see you dropping pounds and feeling better right before their very eyes! By announcing it publicly, you reinforce your own decision and hold yourself accountable. Who knows, you may even inspire your friends and family to follow the path to longevity.

STEP 4: Don't give up!

One of the best motivators will be the fact that eating this way helps you feel better about yourself because you lose weight naturally and have more energy to do the things that make you happy. It will happen literally, overnight. Maybe not in just one day, but within a few days you will most definitely notice a difference. I challenge you to give it just 10 days. In the back of this book, I have provided you with some recipes to get you started on the road to a healthier, happier you. There are specific directions on what to throw out and what to buy at your grocery store. Challenge yourself, you can do anything for just 10 days. Allow your own body to take itself to a deeper level and convince itself of it's true needs. Most importantly, if you cheat on yourself, don't get discouraged. Just start again. Once you get used to your new way of eating, you will feel so much better that you will have little or no desire to go back to your old habits.

STEP 5: Evaluate.

After 2 weeks, go back and evaluate how the new choices you made about food have brought about positive changes within your body and mind. You'll see how these small steps become so important to your life, your love, and your career. These little changes are what build the foundation to better health. Maybe it's something as simple as having regularity or more energy, or maybe you'll notice something much more profound, like the fact that you don't get sick as often as you used to because your cells, the building blocks of life, are strengthened by the pure food.

Whatever changes you notice will help reinforce that you've officially begun the journey toward a lifetime of health and happiness.

I promise you will find wisdom and gratification in knowing that your newly discovered knowledge about nutrition will empower you to make the right choices for yourself and your family, especially if someone you love is in heaven. That someone will bring a little bit of heaven into your home each time you make a good choice about how to nourish your body. When you have the enthusiasm and the passion, you figure out how to achieve your goals.

Are you inspired yet? Perfect! Go clean out your fridge. Together, we will succeed in living healthier, happier lives....producing healthier, happier babies, and leaving our environment a sustainable place to exist for the next millennium.

True beauty emanates.
~ Kate Murray

QUESTIONS AND COMMENTS

The rest of the resources at the back of the book include a seasonal vegetable chart, healthier substitutions for basic food items that you eat every day and are staples in mainstream cooking and baking such as eggs and milk, as well as important guidelines to keep yourself and your kids on the right track to good health.

Now that you've heard my story, I want to hear yours. What prompted you to buy this book and will you pass it on or buy a copy for a friend? Are you interested in sharing a favorite recipe? Do you have more questions?

Please visit my blog to share your story! Also, be sure to flip the pages to find more inspiration including recipes, charts, and additional resources to help you on the path to wellness.

http://asilentcure.org/blog

PART V:
RESOURCES

THE REPLACEMENT CHART

Ready to clean out your fridge and your pantry? Use this chart to find healthier substitutions for foods and ingredients that you consume on a daily basis. I do provide reference to some brand names in this section. That doesn't mean there are not other brands out there on the market, these are simply the ones that I use personally.

Mainstream: Milk (Dairy Milk, from a cow)
Substitution: Almond Milk or Rice Milk

Notes: Almond milk is made from nuts and water, as the name suggests, and Rice Milk is made from rice and water. Almond milk generally comes in sweetened and unsweetened, as well as both vanilla and chocolate. Use unsweetened for your breakfast cereal, or for any recipe that calls for dairy milk because it resembles dairy milk the most. Choose vanilla or chocolate if you are making your own smoothie or "milk shake" for a sweeter taste. If you are concerned about losing weight, do not drink large amounts of nut milk because remember, nuts are still nuts! 2 oz of unsweetened nut milk in your cereal is not going to make you fat, but 16 oz a day as your beverage of choice is. Stick to water when you're thirsty.

Mainstream: Yogurt (Dairy, Greek, etc.)
Substitution: Amande Almond Milk Yogurt

Notes: This particular brand is the most similar in texture, taste, and consistency to dairy yogurt, but since it is made with nut milk, there is obviously no dairy. You'll typically find it in the organic section of your grocery store.

Mainstream: Canola Oil
Substitution: Unsweetened Applesauce or Pumpkin Puree

Notes: This recommendation is mostly for baking...and bonus if you pick apples and make your own applesauce! Unsweetened applesauce works really well in place of oil for many recipes including muffins, cakes, and breads. You can also make your own pumpkin puree, find that recipe in the recipe section at the back of this book.

Mainstream: Olive Oil
Substitution: Braggs Aminos or Vegetable Broth

Notes: Braggs amino acid comes in a bottle that resembles a condiment bottle. It is usually found in the organic section, near the soy sauce and other like condiments. Use the Braggs or vegetable broth in pace of olive oil when sautéing savory dishes on the stovetop or roasting in the oven.

Mainstream: Eggs
Substitution: Ripe, mashed bananas or Ground Flax Seeds or Ground Chia Seeds

Notes: Eggs are typically used as a binder in baking. You can accomplish almost the same thing with mashed bananas or ground flax seeds. Do not be fooled by egg substitutes or egg "whites". The white part of the egg is actually the part that contains the highest concentration of the animal casein.

Mainstream: Potato Chips or Tortilla Chips
Substitution: Baked Vegetable Chips or Baked Pita Bread

Notes: The easiest way to accomplish making your own chips without oil is to use a parchment paper lined baking sheet with whatever you happen to slice on your mandolin. Zucchini, apples, or beets works very well. You can also use a dehydrator. The best part is, you control the ingredients, so you can bake it without oil. Sprinkle cinnamon on apple chips or a pinch of sea salt on zucchini chips. You're going for crunch here, and I know what you're thinking. Don't write off the beet chips until you actually try them. You just might surprise yourself.

Mainstream: Sour Cream Based Dips
Substitution: Hummus

Notes: Use hummus as a base for any type of dip, spinach, vegetable, roasted pepper, or eggplant. You don't have to limit yourself to chic peas either, use any white bean or even lentils as your base, soak, rinse, and puree in a food processor.

Mainstream: Bread, Bagels and English Muffins
Substitution: Food for Life, Alvarado Street (or any brand) Sprouted & Whole Grain Breads, Bagels and English Muffins

Notes: These are usually found in your grocer's freezer section of the organic aisle. The Food For Life and Alvarado Street brands make whole grain and sprouted grain breads and muffins which are much better than the refined grains in traditional english muffins and 99% of all bread in the bread aisle. I like their cinnamon raisin toast.

Mainstream: Pretzels
Substitution: Unique Sprouted Grain Pretzels and "Shells"

Notes: Processed foods still are not the best choice, but the "better" choice is a whole grain pretzel with very few ingredients. Snyders of Hanover also makes a whole grain pretzel, but I'm a little partial to Unique or Sturgis' brands since I live in the pretzel capital of the world.

Mainstream: Breakfast cereals 90% of them
Substitution: Barbara's, Nature's Path, Cascadian Farms brands of breakfast cereal

Notes: It's not even a question of fruit loops anymore when Special K isn't any better. There isn't really an explanation necessary after you look at the ingredient label. We are bombarded with commercials for cereals that pose as the healthier alternative, and then they use Enriched Flour as their first ingredient, followed by a GMO. Yikes.

Mainstream: Fig Newtons and Cereal Bars
Substitution: Barbara's Fig Bars and Cereal Bars

Notes: Again, remember, this is still a processed food, but I like that this brand uses whole grains as a base well as organic fruit.

Mainstream: Popcorn
Substitution: Freshly popped organic popcorn

Notes: Do not use oil, butter, or salt, instead, use a spice. Genetically Modified Corn (GMO) is a big, big issue. Make sure you buy organic corn and popcorn.

Mainstream: Salad dressings with oil
Substitution: Infused Balsamic Vinegar

Notes: This is so much easier than you thought possible. Choose an infused balsamic and then you really don't need any other topping on your salad. Or, to make your own salad dressings, use: Red Wine Vinegar, Champagne Vinegar, Rice Vinegar, Cider Vinegar, or Lemon, Lime, or Grapefruit Juice. Combine with Olives, Tahini, Soy Sauce, Mustard, Capers, Jalapeno, Citrus Zest, or Fresh Ginger. Add fruit and herbs of choice. No oil necessary!

Mainstream: Juice boxes like Capri Sun
Substitution: Honest Kids brand juice pouches

Notes: Yes, it's still juice, but this is the only one on the market that is certified organic and also contains significantly less junk than the other juice boxes out there. From the makers of Honest Tea. Remember, kids come with a warranty. I give my kids a juice pouch in moderation. That means, once every now and then at a party…not twice a day.

Mainstream: Peanut Butter
Substitution: Smuckers "Natural" Peanut Butter

Notes: Most peanut butter contains partially hydrogenated oil as the second ingredient after peanuts. To eliminate the oil, choose the "natural" kind that has just peanuts and salt. The natural peanut oil doe separate, it is normal. Using a spatula, scoop out all peanut butter and oil into a mixing bowl. Whisk it all together, and transfer back into the jar. Refrigerate the jar. It holds up quite well after you mix it.

Mainstream: Ice Cream
Substitution: Homemade Smoothie, Frozen Sorbet, or a Yonanna "Ice Cream" Maker

Notes: While it still contains sugar, at least the commercial brands of sorbet in your grocer's freezer doesn't have dairy. For the creamy consistency of ice cream, substitute the almond milk yogurt in your homemade smoothie. Another way to add creaminess is to use the yonanna with frozen fruit and add avocado to get the smooth consistency. Refer to the smoothie recipes at the back of the book when you are craving either fruit or chocolate in a creamy frozen version.

Mainstream: Ice Tea
Substitution: Freshly brewed, unsweetened, any variety

Notes: I'm a big tea fan, hot or cold. I get this rebuttal almost every time...and the answer is: You can train yourself to drink tea without sweetener, I swear, and once you do, all sweet teas will taste awful to you. Whether you choose green or black, caffeinated or decaf depends on your preference but I love tea and it is my go-to beverage if I crave something besides water.

THE EAT SEASONABLY CHART

Vegetable	Month in Season
Asparagus	April - June
Snap Beans	July - October
Lima Beans	July - October
Beets	July - December
Broccoli	July and July, September to November
Brussels Sprouts	September to December
Cabbage	June to December
Cantaloupe	July to September
Carrots	July to December
Cauliflower	June to July and September to November
Celery	June to February
Sweet Corn	July to October
Cucumber	July - September
Eggplant	July to October
Leaf Lettuce	May to October (Field) Year-Round (Greenhouse)
Peas	May to June
Peppers	July to October
Potatoes	August to March
Pumpkin	September to December
Spinach	May to June and September to October
Summer Squash	June to October
Winter Squash	September to December
Tomatoes	July to October (Field) and April to July, October to December (Greenhouse)
Turnips	August - February
Watermelon	July - October

Notes about the Eat Seasonably Chart:

This eat seasonably calendar is for the state of Pennsylvania. You can find a seasonable food guide for any state in the United States and Canada at this link: http://eatwellguide.org

The source for this information is the Eat Well Guide to local, sustainable, organic produce from GRACE Communications Foundation, New York, NY. Among other environmental and sustainable initiatives, the Eat Well Guide strives to create and promote prevention techniques that individuals and communities can use to improve their health.

For more information:
GRACE Communications Foundation
215 Lexington Avenue, Suite 1001
New York, NY 10016
http://gracelinks.org

Making Sense of Sweeteners

Quite possibly, an entire book could be written about sweeteners. If the dangers of artificial sweeteners are not already blatantly obvious, just Google the term aspartame and you'll see a laundry list of safety concerns that will make you sick, fat, and unfortunately, yes, nearly dead.

Aspartame hides behind brands like NutraSweet, and Equal, but in my opinion, other so-called "naturally occurring" sweeteners like Stevia and Splenda are just as dangerous. Sweetener is not a health food. Many people, especially diabetics, are concerned about the glycemic index. The answer to that is complex. The information below should not be used in place of specific medical advice, but rather as a general guideline for otherwise healthy people.

Sugar supplies energy in the body in the form of glucose, which is the preferred energy source for the brain, central nervous system, and even the placenta; it is the only energy source for red blood cells. With that said, all sweeteners should be used in moderation, and when I use the term moderation, I use it sparingly because everyone has a different definition of moderation.

The USDA recommends that sugar be no more than 5% of your daily intake of calories. Translation? 1 teaspoon of sugar in your coffee is enough added sugar for the whole day. Keep that in mind.

For a larger, printable version of the sweetener chart go to:

http://asilentcure.org/sweetnerchart.pdf

The Sweetener Chart

Sweetener	Best Use	The Science
Table Sugar	Cookies	50% glucose 50% fructose. White sugar has been processed, so there are no minerals or antioxidants.
Xylitol	Cookies, Coffee	Looks and feels like sugar, but contains 40% less food energy and is absorbed more so it prevents high blood sugar spikes.
Agave	Smoothies	Contains up to 90% fructose, the most of any sweetener. Use sparingly in your ice tea or smoothie.
Honey	Salad Dressing or Slaw	Slightly more fructose than glucose, but has antioxidants as well.
Molasses	BBQ Sauce	About the same glucose/fructose as sugar at 50/50, highest antioxidant level and has a distinctly sweet/bitter flavor.
Brown Sugar	Cookies and Cakes	50/50 glucose/fructose just like table sugar, but made by adding molasses back to white sugar. Trace amount of some minerals.
Raw Sugar (Turbinado)	Toppings on Sweets	50/50 glucose/fructose, brown because not all molasses has been stripped out.
Pure Maple Syrup	Salad Dressing and Breakfast	50/50 glucose/fructose with small amounts of antioxidants
Date Sugar	Bar Cookies	Made from ground dates, this delivers all the nutrients of dates such as potassium and is similar in antioxidants to molasses
Coconut Sugar	Use coconut instead.	Made from the sap of the coconut flower, and not a sustainable ingredient. Once the sap has been taken to make sugar, the tree can no longer produce coconuts. Don't use it.

THE RULES OF FOOD COMBINING[16]

1. Sub acid fruits should be combined with acid fruits or sweet fruits.

2. Do not combine acid fruits with sweet fruits.

3. Melons should be eaten alone. The melon is the fastest digesting food. If you eat a meal and then have a few slices of watermelon for dessert, then the watermelon will immediately digest and leave the rest of the meal to rot in your stomach, causing bloating, fullness, and fatigue. Fruits, especially the melons contain simple carbohydrates (sugars) which monopolize all digestive functions so the other foods have to wait and ferment. All melon (watermelon, honeydew, cantaloupe, etc.) should be eaten alone, without any other foods. Think 2:00 pm snack in the middle of the day. You should not eat anything else after eating a melon for at least 2 hours.

4. Do not combine acids and carbohydrates. In other words, do not drink orange juice with toast or cereal. Non-starchy vegetables and ocean vegetables go with anything: proteins, oils and butter, grains, starchy vegetables, lemons and limes. Think raw carrots with hummus, or collard greens sautéed in olive oil with salt and pepper.

5. Do not combine high protein (meat, fish, eggs, cheese) with starch (potato, pasta, bread, cereal) at the same meal. Proteins require acid for their digestion in the stomach, while carbohydrates require alkaline for digestion in the small intestine. Sugars inhibit the secretion of the hydrochloric acid in the stomach and combine with the free hydrochloric acid which interferes with the digestion of proteins. Conversely, if proteins are

189

being digested in the stomach and there is more acid there for the sugar to combine with, then it will require much more alkaline secretion from the pancreas to neutralize the extra acid before it goes to work on the sugar. So what exactly does this mean? Avoid spaghetti and meatballs! For a healthier pasta dish, combine with eggplant and zucchini.

6. All meat, milk, dairy, and eggs should be avoided (except mother's milk for infants). I know, this is a tough one. If you are healthy to begin with, you can start by cutting back; use a *minimal amount* of meat and dairy. If you have already been diagnosed or pre-diagnosed for disease…then obviously the recommendation is to cut out all meat and dairy.

7. Lettuce and celery are commonly thought to aid in the digestion of other foods. Ideally, you should eat a salad at the end of your meal rather than the beginning because the vegetables and presumably vinegar in the salad dressing will aid in the digestion of the starch and protein.

8. Be very careful and conscious of what children eat. A child's digestive system is very delicate, and many chronic diseases later in life including emotional and behavioral problems are the result of too much sugar, salt, fat, and processed food.

How to "Fix It"

- If you eat protein and starch during the same meal, for goodness sake, eat more vegetables!
- If you eat nuts, eat an acid fruit with them.
- If you still eat meat and dairy, eat it with an acid fruit such as pineapple.
- If you ate too much sugar, eat grapes.
- If you ate too much salt, eat watermelon.

Toxicity

According to the Center for Disease Control and Prevention, there are over 80,000 chemicals registered in the U.S., and hundreds of these chemicals are present in our body. Research has shown that these toxins cause imbalance in our endocrine, immune, nervous and reproductive systems. External toxins include air and water pollutants, caffeine, secondhand smoke, household cleaning products, pesticides, herbicides, cosmetics, preservatives, and pharmaceutical medication to name but a few. Take this quiz to determine whether you have exposed yourself to toxicity unknowingly.

The Toxicity Quiz

Yes	No	Do you drink alcohol regularly?
Yes	No	Do you drink coffee regularly?
Yes	No	Do you drink soda regularly? (Doesn't matter, regular/diet)
Yes	No	Do you drink tap water?
Yes	No	Do you eat any processed foods?
Yes	No	Do you eat fruits and vegetables that are not organic?
Yes	No	Do you eat meat and fish?
Yes	No	Do you eat out regularly?
Yes	No	Do you grill foods?
Yes	No	Do you use artificial sweetener?
Yes	No	Have you consumed genetically altered food?
Yes	No	Have you eaten food that contain any dyes or additives?

Notes about the Toxicity Quiz:

If your answers were mostly yes, it should be an eye opener to the amount of toxicity that we really do have some control over. Your internal organs, such as the liver, kidneys, and intestines contribute significantly to the body's ability to rid itself of these toxins. A whole foods, plant-based diet delivers powerful antioxidant protection and supplies the body with amino acids, essential fatty acids and other vitamins to support intestinal, muscular, and immune health.

Source: Centers for Disease Control and Prevention. *Fourth National Report on Human Exposure to Environmental Chemicals*. Atlanta (GA): CDC, 2009, updated tables, 2012. http://www.cdc.gov/exposurereport/

THE CLEAN 15™

VS.

THE MOST PESTICIDE LADEN

	Dirty Dozen		**The Clean 15**
1	Apples	1	Onions
2	Celery	2	Sweet Corn
3	Sweet bell peppers	3	Pineapples
4	Peaches	4	Avocado
5	Strawberries	5	Cabbage
6	Nectarines - imported	6	Sweet Peas
7	Grapes	7	Asparagus
8	Spinach	8	Mangoes
9	Lettuce	9	Eggplant
10	Cucumbers	10	Kiwi
11	Blueberries - domestic	11	Cantaloupe - domestic
12	Potatoes	12	Sweet Potatoes
		13	Grapefruit
		14	Watermelon
		15	Mushrooms

Plus: Green beans, Kale/Greens (many contain residues of special concern.) Source: ewg.org

Headquartered in Washington, DC, the Environmental Working Group (EWG) is a team of scientists, engineers, policy experts, lawyers and computer programmers that uses government data, legal documents, scientific studies and their own laboratory tests to expose threats to public health and the environment, and to find solutions.

RECIPES

All of these recipes have been developed by me (except where noted) with luxurious, plant-based ingredients and copious care. They come to you straight from my kitchen to yours. I take great pride in the fact that I am a "cook-from-scratch" entertainer, and I go to great lengths to test my recipes over and over to make sure the flavor combinations are just right. There are many substitutions out there, but if you follow the recipe, it will produce a delicious and healthy result.

Please note that while these recipes are generally very low-fat, plant-based and healthy, my recipes alone are not a diet prescription. If you suffer from any type of disease or health condition, you should *absolutely consult with a qualified medical practitioner.* But hey, at least you know what kinds of questions to ask now! Vegan meal preparation is not easy; different flavor combinations produce different results, different types of flour produce different textures, and leavening agents such as baking soda and baking powder do matter and are not interchangeable. If I could simply publish my last decade of recipes, I have no doubt they would be delectable, but at the same time, not nearly as healthy as I would like them to be. On the horizon? A recipe book... after a few more years of dedicated experimentation. Why? I want it to be exquisite! I don't want it to be one of those cookbooks in which only 2 out of 50 recipes are actually good ones. You have my promise, all of the recipes will be simply divine.

In the meantime, check my recipe blog often for the latest recipes and wellness inspiration.

Risotto
w/Mushroom, Onion, & Asparagus

Makes 4-6 Servings

Ingredients

2 Cups Arborio Rice
1 Large Vidalia Onion
1 Cup Sliced Baby Portobello Mushrooms
1 Cup Crimini Mushrooms
6 Cups Vegetable Broth
1 Cup Dry Marsalla Cooking Wine
1 Bunch of Asparagus
Salt & Pepper

Toast the rice in a skillet (begin by coating the bottom with about 1/2 cup of vegetable broth to prevent sticking) on your stovetop on medium heat until translucent, about 5 minutes. Add vegetable broth, about a cup at at time, mixing frequently. It's better if the broth is heated. Once the rice soaks up the broth, continue adding, a cup at a time. Once you've added about 4 cups of broth, add the Marsalla for the next one. Continue in this manner until the rice is cooked.

In between stirring your risotto, give your onions and mushrooms a rough chop. Then, in a separate skillet, sauté onions and mushrooms with salt and pepper, until caramelized. Add the onion and mushrooms mixture to the rice skillet. I like to sauté the onions and mushrooms separately because it interferes with my rice toasting. You can do it all together if you choose.

Chop the asparagus into about 1 inch segments, and add it right at the end. Cover and allow the asparagus to stem lightly, it should be aldente, a slight crunch, but not crispy.

Butternut Squash Lasagna

Ingredients

Tbsp. Braggs Aminos
1 Large Vidalia Onion
2 Cloves of Garlic
10 Cups Organic Greens (Spinach, Kale, or Swiss Chard)
1 Medium Butternut Squash, Peeled and Cubed
Lasagna Noodles (Regular, No Boil, Brown Rice Noodles, etc.)
Vegan "Ricotta Cheese" (See Recipe Below)
6 Cups Organic Tomato Sauce (Jarred or Make Your Own)
1 tsp. Coriander
Salt & Pepper

Vegan "Ricotta Cheese" Ingredients

1 lb. Extra Firm Tofu, well drained
1 tsp. Lemon Juice
1/4 Cup Nutritional Yeast
1/4 tsp. Garlic Powder
Salt and Pepper
Toss with your fingers until crumbled, then combine with greens.

Squash Preparation: Roast cleaned, cubed squash with salt and pepper at 425 for about 20 minutes or until fork tender.

Greens Preparation: Sauté onions with a small amount of Braggs, until caramelized. Add crushed garlic at the very end; sauté 1 more minute. Transfer to a food processor. In the same skillet, sauté cleaned, de-stemmed greens (add more Braggs if necessary) for 2 minutes, until the color becomes dark and slightly wilted. Add greens to onion mixture and pulse until coarsely chopped.

Assembly: Layer noodles, greens/ricotta, sauce, noodles, squash, noodles, sauce. Repeat layers in the same order. Bake at 375 for about 45 minutes. Be sure to fully coat noodles with sauce otherwise they will get hard.

Potato & Celery Root "Au Gratin"

Makes 4-6 Servings

Ingredients

4 Large Shallots, Sliced Thin
Salt & Pepper
2 Celery Roots, Peeled and Sliced Thin
3-4 lbs. Russet or Golden Potatoes, Peeled and Sliced Thin
1 Cup Vegetable Broth
1-2 Cups Almond Milk (or other non-dairy milk)
Chopped Fresh Thyme
1 Tbsp. Arrowroot

Preparation Notes: Lightly spray the bottom of a baking dish. Layer shallots, then celery root, then potatoes, sprinkle salt, pepper, and thyme. Repeat the layering.

Bring the almond milk and broth to a boil over medium high heat, add arrowroot, stirring frequently until thicker.

Pour over the vegetables and bake at 400 degrees, covered, for about 30-40 minutes. Remove foil and sprinkle chopped thyme over the top. Bake uncovered another 5-10 minutes or until the edges of the gratin are golden brown.

Burritos w/Guacamole

Makes 6-8 Servings

Ingredients

1 tsp. Braggs Liquid Aminos
1 Large Vidalia Onion, Roughly Chopped
Salt & Pepper
4 Cloves of Garlic, Minced
1 Zucchini, Roughly Chopped
1 Red Bell Pepper
2 Cups of Black Beans, Rinsed and Soaked (or 1 can, rinsed)
2 Cups of Pinto Beans, Rinsed, Soaked, Mashed (or 1 can)
Chopped Kale
Ezekiel or another Whole Grain Wrap

Use the Braggs to coat the bottom of a skillet, and sauté onions with salt and pepper on medium high until translucent. Turn down the heat to medium, add garlic, and sauté for another minute. Add zucchini and sauté for another 5 minutes. Add black beans and kale to mixture, then add the mashed pintos and combine well to form a paste. Turn the heat off immediately.

Fill the wraps with the mixture, roll up the burritos and bake in the oven for 10 minutes at 300 degrees. Can be served warm or at room temperature with a side of guacamole. (Guacamole recipe follows.)

Guacamole

Serve with baked pita chips or as a condiment for burritos

Ingredients

4 Ripe Avocados
1/2 Small Red Onion
1/2 Cup Chopped Parsley or Cilantro
1-2 tsp. Tobasco Sauce
Juice of 1 Lemon
Sea Salt & Freshly Ground Black Pepper

I like to puree two of the avocados with red onion so you get the flavor without biting into a raw onion. I mash the other two avocados to get both a creamy and chunky consistency.

Acorn Squash Filled w/Lentils

Makes 6 Servings

Ingredients

3 Acorn Squash
1 Tbsp. Braggs Liquid Aminos
Salt & Freshly Ground Black Pepper

For the filling:

1/2 Cup Dry Lentils
1/2 Cup White Wine
1/2 Cup Water
1/2 Cup Capers (plus 2 tbsp. juice)
1/2 Cup Stuffed Olives, (Manzanillas) plus 2 tbsp. juice
1 Cup Dried Prunes, Roughly Chopped (approximately 25)
1/4 Cup Brown Sugar

Step 1: Slice the squash in half and scoop out the seeds and stringy filling. Brush each half with Braggs, sprinkle salt and pepper, and roast on a baking sheet, sliced side up, at 400 degrees for 20 minutes.

Step 2: Bring the water and wine to a boil and add lentils. Reduce the heat to low, cover, and cook for about 15 minutes or until the lentils are tender.

Once the lentils are al'dente, add them to the rest of the filling and stir gently. Fill the squash and put it back in the oven. Turn the heat down to 350 degrees, and bake for about 20-30 more minutes or until the flesh of the squash is fork tender.

This recipe makes a great entertaining dish!

Chard & Sweet Potato Fritters
w/Ginger Lime Dipping Sauce

Makes 4-6 Servings

Ingredients

2 Cups Rinsed and Soaked or 1 Can of Cannelloni Beans
2 Cups Rinsed and Soaked or 1 Can of Chic Peas
3-4 Cups Swiss Chard
1/2 Cup Nutritional Yeast
2 Medium Sweet Potatoes
2 Cups Panko Bread Crumbs
1/2 Tsp. Paprika
1/2 Tsp. Coriander
1/2 Tsp. Nutmeg

Peal and chop the sweet potatoes, roast or boil until fork tender. Pulse cannelloni beans, sweet potato, spices and nutritional yeast in a food processor until a chunky but pureed consistency.

Chop and lightly steam or sauté the swiss chard until just wilted.

Lightly mash the chic peas, and then fold in the sweet potato mixture, the chard, and half the bread crumbs. Form into patties and coat each patty with more panko bread crumbs.

Bake at 400 degrees for about 15 minutes or until golden.

Serve with the Ginger Lime Dipping Sauce/Salad Dressing

Ginger Lime Dipping Sauce

For best results, combine ingredients in a salad dressing mixer.

Ingredients

Zest and Juice of one Lime

2 Tbsp. Rice Vinegar

1 Tbsp. Ginger root (grated)

1 Clove Garlic (minced)

1 Tbsp. Tamari

1 Tbsp. Honey (or agave nectar, or pure maple syrup)

1 Tbsp. Dijon Mustard

1 tsp. Sugar (or Honey or Agave)

Maple Hazelnut Brussels Sprouts

Makes 4-6 Servings

Ingredients

1/2 - 3/4 Cup Hazelnuts, lightly toasted, skin removed
4-6 Cups of Brussels Sprouts (about half a stalk)
1 Small Red Onion
1/4 Cup Maple Syrup
2 tsp. Apple Cider Vinegar

Toast hazelnuts until fragrant, and rub off skin with a kitchen towel. Chop coarsely and set aside.

Half Brussels and loosely chop the onion, sprinkle with salt and pepper, and roast uncovered on a sprayed baking sheet at 425 for about 20-30 minutes or until edges are slightly browned.

Combine maple syrup and vinegar in a bowl and drizzle over the top, roast for about 5 more minutes and toss chopped hazelnuts on top.

Quinoa Citrus Salad

Ingredients

4 Cups Quinoa
2 Mangoes
1 Whole Pineapple
2 Cucumbers
2 Cups Fresh Chopped Parsley
Salt & Pepper
Citrus Vinaigrette (Recipe Follows)

Prepare quinoa according to package directions and allow to cool.

Dice the mangoes and pineapple. Scrub cucumber, slice in half and remove the seedy middle. Sprinkle with salt and allow to drain for about 30 minutes. Wipe excess water off the cucumber and dice.

Once quinoa is moderately cool, top with diced fruits and veggies, salt and pepper, and then toss with citrus dressing. Chill for a few hours or overnight to allow flavors to blend together. The best part about this salad is that it holds up well at a summer picnic.

Citrus Vinaigrette

For best results, combine with a salad dressing mixer

Ingredients

Juice and Zest of 1 Grapefruit, 1 Orange, & 1 Lemon
1 Tbsp. Champagne Vinegar
2 Tsp. Sugar (or Honey or Agave)
2 Tbsp. Dijon Mustard
1 Tbsp. Freshly Chopped Oregano
1 Tbsp. Freshly Chopped Basil
Salt & Freshly Ground Black Pepper

Seductive Cranberry Slaw

Ingredients

Full Head of Red Cabbage, Shredded
Fresh Apples (any variety) Cored and Julienned (skin on)
Juice of 1 Lemon (to coat apples after you julienne them)
1 Cup Dried Cranberries
1 Cup Chopped Walnuts, Lightly Toasted

Dressing

1/3 Cup Rice Vinegar
1/3 Cup Champagne Vinegar
2 Tbsp. Sugar
Salt & Freshly Ground Black Pepper

Toss cabbage, apples, and cranberries together in a large bowl. Prepare dressing with a salad dressing mixer for best results and then pour dressing over the mixture. Toss to combine and then top with chopped walnuts.

Asparagus & White Bean Salad w/Raspberry Vinaigrette

Makes 4-6 Servings

Ingredients

1 Bunch of Asparagus
1 Cup Soaked (or about 1/2 a can rinsed) Navy Beans
1 Small Red Onion, Sliced Thin
4-6 Cups Baby Spinach
2-4 Cups Arugula
2 Cups Grape Tomatoes
1 Cup Walnuts, Lightly Toasted

Use a vegetable peeler to ribbon the asparagus. Layer the spinach, arugula, onion, asparagus, navy beans, then walnuts, in that order. Drizzle with Raspberry Vinaigrette.

Raspberry Vinaigrette

For best results, combine in a salad dressing mixer

Ingredients

1 Small Shallot
2 Tbsp. Dijon Mustard
2 Tbsp. Tarragon Vinegar
2 Tsp. Sugar (or Honey or Agave)
1 Tsp. Chambord or Raspberry Liqueur
1/2 Tsp. Garlic Salt
4-5 Fresh or Frozen Raspberries
Freshly Chopped Parsley (or 1 Tbsp. Dried)
Freshly Chopped Tarragon (or 1 Tbsp. Dried)
Freshly Ground Black Pepper

CARROT RADISH SALAD
w/PEANUT DRESSING

Serves 6-8

INGREDIENTS

3 lbs. Carrots, Cleaned & Peeled
1/2 Head of Green Japanese Cabbage
1 Bunch Radishes
Salt & Freshly Ground Black Pepper

Julienne the carrots and cabbage. Slice the radishes thin; for best results, use a mandolin. Toss with Peanut Dressing. Serve cold or at room temperature.

PEANUT SALAD DRESSING

For best results, use a salad dressing mixer.

INGREDIENTS

1/2 Cup Natural Peanut Butter
2 Tbsp. Rice Vinegar
2 Tbsp. Tamari or Soy Sauce
2 tsp. Sugar (or Honey or Agave)
Juice and Zest of 1 Lemon
2 Tbsp. Freshly Grated Ginger
1/4 tsp. Cayenne (optional for kick)
1 Clove Garlic (minced)
Toasted Sesame Seeds (optional)

CREAMY POTATO SALAD

Serves 8-10

INGREDIENTS

3-5 lbs. Small New Potatoes, Skin on
1 cup of Plain Non-dairy Yogurt (such as Amande), Strained
1/4 Cup of Non-dairy Milk (such as almond milk)
2 Tbsp. Dijon Mustard
2 Tbsp. Grainy Mustard
1 Cup Chopped Celery
1/2 Cup Finely Chopped Red Onion
1/2 Cup Chopped Fresh Dill
Kosher Salt & Freshly Ground Black Pepper

Cube potatoes (keep the skin on) and boil or steam until fork tender. Be careful not to over-cook the potatoes, the skin should not come off. Strain the non-dairy yogurt so it's not watery. I use a colander with a paper towel inside of it, then place the yogurt in the colander. Put the colander in the fridge for at least an hour to strain. Discard the yogurt water. It is essential to strain the yogurt, otherwise, the dressing will be watery instead of creamy.

While potatoes are still cooking, chop the celery and dice the red onion. Once the yogurt is strained, transfer to a large mixing bowl and add remaining ingredients; whisk together to form a sauce. Drain the potatoes. When the potatoes are cool, add the celery and onion. Then, pour the sauce over everything; cover and refrigerate for several hours to allow the flavors to combine.

Wild Rice Salad
w/Lemon Dijon Dressing

Serves 6-8

Ingredients

4 Cups Wild Rice, Cooked and Drained
2 Cups Tiny Peas, Cooked
2 Cups Baby Portobello Mushrooms, Sliced
4 Green Onions, Sliced Thin
Kosher Salt & Freshly Ground Black Pepper

Combine all ingredients and drizzle with Creamy Italian
Vinaigrette (Recipe Follows).

Lemon Dijon Dressing

For Best Results, use a Salad Dressing Mixer

Ingredients

Juice and Zest of 1 Lemon
1/4 Cup Unsweetened Almond Milk
1 Tbsp. Dijon Mustard
2 tsp. Sugar or Agave
1/4 Cup White Balsamic Vinegar
2 tsp. Freshly Chopped Basil (or Dried Basil)
1 tsp. Freshly Chopped Oregano (or Dried Oregano)
Salt & Freshly Ground Black Pepper

Black Bean & Corn Salad

Serves 6-8

Ingredients

4 Cups Black Beans, Soaked/Rinsed (or 2 Cans, Rinsed)
4-6 Ears of Corn, Steamed, Cooled, and Cut off the Stalk
2 lbs. Organic Celery, Scrubbed, Peeled and Diced
1/4 Cup Freshly Chopped Parsley

Be sure to use organic celery, it's one of the Dirty Dozen. Also, be sure to use fresh, non-GMO corn for best results. Canned corn just isn't the same!

Toss with Basic Vinaigrette (recipe follows).

This salad is quite versatile; it can be used as a stand-alone side salad, added to a wrap with spinach for a lunch, or used as a "dip" with tortilla chips.

Basic Vinaigrette

For best results, use a salad dressing mixer.

Ingredients

Juice and Zest of 1 Lemon
1 Tbsp. Dijon Mustard
2 tsp. Sugar (or Honey or Agave)
1/4 Cup White Vinegar
2 Tbsp. Freshly Chopped Basil (or Dried Basil)
1 Tbsp. Freshly Chopped Oregano (or Dried Oregano)
Salt & Freshly Ground Black Pepper

My Favorite Lunch Wrap

The ultimate "go-to" and "on-the-go" lunch!

Ingredients

Whole Grain Wrap
1 Tbsp. Hummus
Organic Baby Spinach Leaves
Broccoli Sprouts
1 Radish, Sliced Thin
Cucumber Slices, Thin, About 5 Slices
Chopped Celery
Carrot Ribbons (use a vegetable peeler)

I always keep the above veggies in our fridge, so this is my go-to wrap for lunch. Easy and filling! Experiment with other raw veggies in there too like slices of bell peppers, green beans, snap peas, and avocado.

CARLA COLADA

For best results, use a Vitamix

INGREDIENTS

1/2 of a Pineapple, Peeled and Cubed
1 Mango, Peeled and Cubed
1 Cup Low-fat Coconut Milk (I like Silk Pure Coconut Milk)
1 Cup Rice Milk
2 Cups Crushed Ice

Really, that's it. Combine ingredients in a Vitamix or a food processor. Coconut milk *is not low-fat*, so use this recipe as a treat once in a while, not an everyday staple.

JOE'S CHOCO SQUAD

For best results, use a Vitamix

INGREDIENTS

2 Frozen Bananas
1 Cup Unsweetened Oats
1 Tbsp. Ground Flax Seeds
1 Tbsp. Cocoa
2 Cups Unsweetened Almond Milk

Process the oats first into a flour, then add the rest of the ingredients. You can also substitute chocolate almond milk instead of regular almond milk and eliminate the cocoa, but that ups the calories and makes it sweeter. 2 ripe bananas can be substituted with 1 cup of crushed ice if you don't have a banana already frozen. I like to peal and slice my "almost over-ripe" bananas and keep them in the freezer.

Summer Berry Love

Ingredients

1 Cup of Plain Almond Milk Yogurt (I like Amande)
1 Cup Blueberries
1 Cup Strawberries
1 Cup Blackberries
1 Cup Raspberries
1 Tbsp. Raspberry Agave

If the berries are frozen, you won't need ice, if the berries are fresh, I usually add about 1 cup of crushed ice to give it the smoothie consistency rather than a juice consistency.

You can use a berry flavored almond yogurt instead of plain, just eliminate the Agave, you won't need a sweetener because the yogurt is already sweetened.

Strength in Green Smoothie

For best results, use a Vitamix.

Ingredients

1 "Sprig" of Kale
1/4 Cup Fresh Spinach
1 Tbsp. Almonds
2 Tbsp. Dates
1 Tbsp. Maple Syrup
1 tsp. Cinnamon
1 Cup Rice Milk
2 Cups Ice

Blend almonds first, then add kale, spinach and rice milk. Add dates, maple syrup and ice at the end.

Blend to desired consistency and top with another dash of cinnamon.

August Melon Smoothie

For best results, use a Vitamix.

Ingredients

2-3 Cups Chopped Watermelon
1/2 Cup Seltzer Water
2 Cups Ice
2-4 Sprigs of Fresh Mint
Juice of 1 Lime

Blend away! This is a wonderful treat on a hot summer day.

Easy Toast w/PB & Banana

Use on Ezekiel or Whole Grain Toast, English Muffin, or Bagel

Ingredients

1 Slice of Whole Grain Bread, Toasted
1 Banana, Sliced Thin
1 Tbsp. Natural Peanut Butter

Spelt Waffles

You can sub any whole grain, gluten-free flour.

Ingredients

2 Cups Light Spelt Flour
1 Tbsp. Baking Powder
1 Tbsp. Flax Seeds
1 Cup Rice Milk
1 Tbsp. Maple Syrup
1 Ripe Mashed Banana

Blend well. For best results, use a waffle iron.

Topping Ingredients

1/4 Cup Maple Syrup
2 Plain Almond Yogurt
1 Peach, sliced
1/4 Cup Blueberries
Crushed Walnuts

Whisk maple syrup and almond yogurt. Drizzle over the top of the waffles, and then top with crushed walnuts, peaches, and blueberries.

Blackberry & Maple Oatmeal

Use on Whole or Rolled Oats, Unsweetened

Ingredients

1 Cup Oats
1/2 Cup Unsweetened Almond Milk (heated)
1/2 Cup Blackberries
1 Tbsp. Maple Syrup

The combination of the sweet maple syrup with the sour blackberry is out of this world.

English Muffin
w/Fig & Cranberry Jam

Use on Whole Grain Toast, English Muffin, or Bagel

Ingredients

4-5 Fresh Figs, Inside squeezed out (discard skin)
4 Cups Cranberries
1 Cup Water
1 Tbsp. Pectin
1/4 Cup Sugar or Brown Sugar (if desired)

Add the fruit and water to a pot on the stovetop and bring to a boil on medium high, stirring frequently. As the fruit heats up, begin to mash the fruit together. Reduce the heat to low, add remaining ingredients and simmer until desired thickness is reached (about 15 minutes).

Jam keeps for about a week in the refrigerator.

Apricot Bars

You can use apricots, peaches, or nectarines.

Ingredients: Apricot Jam

10-14 Organic Apricots (depends on size) or 4-6 Peaches
1/4 Cup Pectin
2-3 Tbsp. Sugar

Bring to a boil on the stovetop, then reduce the heat and simmer until thick, jam-like consistency. It's better to remove the skin for some fruits (apricots have a thin skin, so I usually don't remove those skins) but for the peaches, I boiled them for several minutes and then put them into an ice bath. Then the thick skin peals right off. It's a bit time consuming, but well worth the effort. I only use 1 tablespoon of sugar because when peaches are ripe and in season, they do not need to be sweetened much more. In a pinch, you can use a jar of organic jam.

Ingredients: Crust

1 Cup Unsweetened Applesauce
1/2 Cup Sugar
2 Tbsp. Ground Flax Seeds
1 Cup Finely Chopped Walnuts
1 Cup Quinoa Flour
1 Cup Brown-Rice Four

Whirl the crust ingredients in a food processor and press firmly into a sprayed 9x11 baking pan. Reserve about 1/2 cup of the crust to sprinkle on the top. Top the crust with the jam, and sprinkle the remaining crust over the top. Bake at 350 degrees for about 35 minutes or until slightly golden brown. Serve as a breakfast or dessert.

Oatmeal Raisin Cookies

Dry Ingredients

2 Cups Rolled Oats
1/2 Cup Light Brown Sugar
1 tsp. Baking Powder
1 Tbsp. Cinnamon
1 Tbsp. Corn Starch
1/2 Cup Raisins

Wet Ingredients

1/3 Cup Unsweetened Applesauce
1 tsp. Vanilla Extract
1/4 Cup Unsweetened Almond Milk

Combine dry ingredients together first. Mix wet ingredients together in a separate bowl, then fold wet into dry until you get a thick, batter-like consistency. Add the raisins last. I use a melon baller to get evenly sized cookies. Line a baking sheet with parchment paper, and dollop each cookie. Press down a bit, they will not expand so you can put them close together.

Bake at 400 for about 10-14 minutes or until golden.

Michelle's Marvelous Applesauce

Thank you Michelle Stout; the kitchen smells delicious!

Ingredients

8-10 Apples, Peeled, Cored, & Sliced
(Cortland, Empire, & Macintosh)
1/2 Cup of Water
1 Tbsp. Cinnamon
1 Tbsp. Grated Orange Zest (optional)
1-2 Tbsp. Sugar or Agave (if desired)

Add all ingredients to a crock pot, cover, and simmer on low for about 6-8 hours. Stir until your desired consistency is reached.

If you use the orange zest, substitute the 1/2 cup of water with the juice of the orange. The flavor really kicks the applesauce up a notch giving it a sweet and sour flavor.

Notes: You can use any variety of apples, but the key to a unique taste is to use a few different varieties of apples. Also, it's most likely that you will not need any additional sweetener at all, especially since some apple varieties are very sweet already.

LISA'S DIVINE CHOCOLATE TORTE

The chocoholic in all of us thanks you, Lisa Banco!

DRY INGREDIENTS:

1 Cup Sprouted Grain Flour
1/3 Cup Unsweetened Cocoa Powder
1 tsp. Baking Soda
1 tsp. Sea Salt
1 Cup Coconut Sugar

Combine all dry ingredients in small bowl and set aside.

WET INGREDIENTS:

1 Cup Unsweetened Chocolate Almond Milk
1 Cup Unsweetened Apple Sauce
1 Tbsp. Pure Vanilla Extract
1 Tbsp. Agave
2 Tbsp. Coconut Vinegar

Combine wet ingredients in food processor. Gradually add dry ingredients to wet.

Bake at 375 degrees in an 8" square or 9" round lightly sprayed baking dish for 18-20 minutes, or until a toothpick inserted comes out clean.

GLAZE:

Melt dark chocolate bar of choice or carob chips over a double boiler. Drizzle over the torte once it is completely cooled.

Spice Muffins

You can sub zucchini for carrot, or no vegetable at all. Yields 20.

Dry Ingredients:

2-3 Carrots (Peeled and Chopped)
1/2 Cup Chopped Almonds
1/2 Cup Golden Raisins

3/4 Cup Brown-Rice Flour
3/4 Cup Quinoa Flour
1 Cup Rolled Oats
1/2 Cup Sugar
1 Tbsp. Baking Powder
1 tsp. Cinnamon
1 tsp. Cloves
1 tsp. Nutmeg
1 Tbsp. Kosher Salt

Wet Ingredients:

1 Cup Pumpkin Pie Spice (recipe follows)
1 Tbsp. Apple Cider Vinegar
1/4 Cup Agave Syrup
Juice and Zest of 1 Orange
1/2 Cup Unsweetened Applesauce

Chop or julienne carrots in a food processor and then remove and set aside. Pulse remaining dry ingredients in the processor next. Combine wet ingredients in a separate mixing bowl and then fold the wet into the dry slowly to combine. Fold in the carrots, raisins, and chopped almonds last. Pour into muffin pan and bake for 20 minutes at 375 degrees or until a toothpick comes out dry. Fill at least 3/4 of each muffin cup.

Homemade Pumpkin Pie Spice

I rarely use anything out of a can.

Dry Ingredients (Spices):

2 tbsp. cup ground cinnamon

2 tbsp. ground ginger

2 tsp. ground cloves

1 tsp. ground nutmeg

1/2 tsp. ground cardamom

Step 1: Wash the exterior of the pumpkin with soap and water.

Step 2: Cut the pumpkin in half with a large chef's knife. You need a large knife because it's not easy to cut through a pumpkin.

Step 3: Scoop out the seeds and scrape the stringy stuff, discard.

Step 4: Remove the stem.

Step 5: Steam or bake in the oven. Steaming on the stovetop will take about 10-15 minutes while baking in the oven takes about 45 minutes to an hour at 375 degrees.

Step 6: Once the inside is tender, you can scoop it out with a spoon, and most of the time, the skin will lift right off. Discard skin.

Step 7: Puree in a food processor with spices.

Step 8: If you want a thicker consistency, you can strain overnight in the fridge.

The pumpkin puree will keep in the fridge for 2-3 days. You can also freeze it. DO NOT try to "can" your own pumpkin puree (or puree from winter squash for that matter). The USDA advises against canning your own at home. For more information, check out the National Center for Home Food Preservation: http://nchfp.uga.edu/tips/fall/pumpkins.html

Notes: It's important to remember that if you "taste" this pumpkin spice when it's finished, it is not going to be very sweet. It is not meant to be sweet because it is a filling that is to be used in other recipes, it is not a "stand-alone" recipe. So don't go eating it like it's cookie dough or you're not going to be very happy after all that work!

ADDITIONAL RESOURCES

The following books are recommended additional reading on the topic of nutrition and disease in no particular order.

The China Study: T. Colin Campbell

Prevent & Reverse Heart Disease: Caldwell B. Esselstyn, Jr., M.D.

Dr. McDougall's Digestive Tune Up: (and various others) John A. McDougall, MD

Keep it Simple, Keep it Whole: Alona Pulde, MD and Matthew Lederman, MD

Breaking the Food Seduction: Neal Barnard, MD

The Devil in the Milk: Keith Woodford

Nutrition and Physical Degeneration, 7th Edition: Weston A. Price DDS

The Whole Soy Story: The Dark Side of America's Favorite Health Food: Kaayla T. Daniel, PhD, CCN

Dr. Dean Ornish's Program for Reversing Heart Disease: The Only System Scientifically Proven to Reverse Heart Disease Without Drugs or Surgery: Dean Ornish

The Engine 2 Diet: Rip Esselstyn

The Best Homemade Babyfood on the Planet: Karin Knight, RN and Tina Ruggiero, MS, RD, LD

The Moss Reports (Many): http://cancerdecisions.com

ABOUT THE AUTHOR

Kate Murray is an avid runner and lives with her husband and children in Shillington, Pennsylvania. She is passionate about educating people about how overall wellness is deeply rooted in proper nutrition. She was practically raised in her mother's kitchen, but it wasn't until she became a mother herself that she realized Americans have such widely varied understandings about what healthy eating really means.

In 2001, she began to focus her attention on nutrition, later focusing very specifically on plant-based nutrition. As a mother, Kate understands the challenges parents face in trying to teach their children to eat more vegetables: "It's not easy when everyone else is serving yogurt and cheese because they think it's the right thing to do."

Kate received her Bachelor's Degree in Communication in 1996 and her Master's of Business Administration in 2003. She also completed a post-graduate certificate in plant based nutrition. Kate is available on a limited basis for lectures, keynote presentations, and workshops about plant-based nutrition.

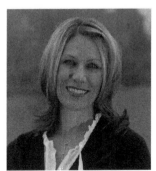

Photo © Ryan McFadden, Reading Eagle

REFERENCES

1. American Cancer Society. *Cancer Facts & Figures 2012*. Atlanta: American Cancer Society; 2012.
http://asilentcure.org/references/CancerFactsFigures2012.pdf

2. Campbell, T.C. (2006). *The China Study: Startling Implications for Diet, Weight Loss, and Long-Term Health.* Dallas, TX: Benbella Books. Link: http://www.thechinastudy.com

3. Lets Eat For the Health of It. USDA Publication number: HHS-ODPHP-2012-01-DGA-B. June, 2011.
Link: http://asilentcure.org/references/USDA_brochure.pdf

4. American Cancer Society. *Cancer Facts & Figures 2011*. Atlanta: American Cancer Society; 2011.
Link: http://asilentcure.org/references/acsfacts2011.pdf

5. The National Center for Biotechnology
Link: http://www.ncbi.nlm.nih.gov/

6. CA: A Cancer Journal for Clinicians. 2012;62:30-67.
Link: http://asilentcure.org/references/acs_guidelines_nutrition2012.pdf

7. Spinach Chart: U.S. Department of Agriculture. "USDA Nutrient Database for Standard Reference." Washington, DC: U.S. Department of Agriculture, Agriculture Research Service, 2002.
http://www.nal.usda.gov/fnic/foodcomp/cgi- bin/nut_search_new.pl

8. Allman-Farinelli, M. A., Gomes, K., Favaloro, E.J., & Petocz, P. (2005). A diet rich in high-oleic-acid sunflower oil favorably alters low-density lipoprotein cholesterol, triglycerides, and factor VII coagulant activity. *American Dietetic Association.Journal of the American Dietetic Association, 105*(7), 1071-1079.
Link: http://asilentcure.org/references/AllmanFarinelli2005.pdf (Note, this is the abstract, not the full article)

9. Anand, P., Kunnumakara, A. B., Sundaram, C., Harikumar, K. B., Tharakan, S. T., Lai, O. S., . . . Aggarwal, B. B. (2008). Cancer is a preventable disease that requires major lifestyle changes. *Pharmaceutical Research, 25*(9), 2097-2116. doi:10.1007/s11095-008-9661-9
http://asilentcure.org/references/cancerprevent.pdf

"Grow It, Cook It, Eat It" at www.rodaleinstitute.org.

10. Uric Acid Level and Elevated Blood Pressure in US Adolescents: National Health and Nutrition Examination Survey, 1999–2006. *Hypertension.* 59:811-817

11. Breastfeeding and the Use of Human Milk. *Pediatrics* 2005;115;496 DOI: 10.1542/peds.2004-2491 http://asilentcure.org/references/breastfeeding.pdf

12. Sellmeyer DE, Stone KL, Sebastian A, et al. "A high ratio of dietary animal to vegetable protein increases the rate of bone loss and the risk of fracture in postmenopausal women." *American Journal of Clinical Nutrition*, 73 (2001): 118–122.

13. Frassetto LA, Todd KM, Morris C, Jr., et al. "World incidence of hip fracture in elderly women relation to consumption of animal and vegetable foods." *Journals of Gerentology* 55 (2000): M585-M592.

14. Onkamo P, Vaananen S, Karvonen M, et al. "Worldwide increase in incidence of Type 1 diabetes—the analysis of the data on published incidence trends." *Diabetologia* 42 (1999): 1395–1403.

15. Karjalainen J, Martin JM, Knip M, et al. "A bovine albumin peptide as a possible trigger of insulin-dependent Diabetes Mellitus." *New Engl. Journ. Med* 327 (1992): 302-307

16. Pitchford, P. (2002) *Healing wih Whole Foods, Third Edition.* Berkley, CA: North Atlantic Books.

17. Leighton, Terrance, Chairman of Microbiology and Immunology at the University of California, Berkeley; press release on "quercetin" in *San Francisco Examiner*, p D-19, Nov. 12, 1989.

18. Lanou AJ, Berkow SE, Barnard ND. Calcium, dairy products, and bone health in children and young adults: a reevaluation of the evidence. *Pediatrics.* 2005;115(3):736-743.

19. Feskanich D, Willett WC, Colditz GA. Calcium, vitamin D, milk consumption, and hip fractures: a prospective study among postmenopausal women. *Am J Clin Nutr.* 2003;77(2):504-511.

20. Esselstyn CB, Ellis SG, Medendorp SV, et al. "A strategy to arrest and reverse coronary artery disease: a 5-year longitudinal study of a single physician's practice." *J. Family Practice* 41 (1995): 560-580.

21. *The Whole Soy Story: The Dark Side of America's Favorite Health Food.* Kaayla T. Daniel, PhD, CCN. (2005) Net Trends Publishing, Washington, DC.

22. Crystal Smith-Spangler, Margaret L. Brandeau, Grace E. Hunter, J. Clay Bavinger, Maren Pearson, Paul J. Eschbach, Vandana Sundaram, Hau Liu, Patricia Schirmer, Christopher Stave, Ingram Olkin, Dena M. Bravata; Are Organic Foods Safer or Healthier Than Conventional Alternatives?A Systematic Review. *Annals of Internal Medicine.* 2012 Sep;157(5):348-366. http://annals.org/article.aspx?articleid=1355685

23.http://www.naturalnews.com/037108_Stanford_Ingram_Olkin_Big_Tob acco.html

24. Popper, A. Pamela. *Solving America's Healthcare Crisis* (2011).

25. Brazier, Brandon and Hugh Jackson. *Thrive: The Vegan Nutrition Guide to Optimal Performance in Sports and Life.* (2008).

26. *Breaking the Food Seduction.* Neal Barnard, M.D. (2003) St. Martin's Press. New York, NY.

27. Woodford, Keith. *Devil in the Milk: Illness, Health and the Politics of A1 and A2 Milk.* (2007). Craig Potton Publishing, Nelson, New Zealand. Printed in the US at First Chelsea green printing, March, 2009.

28.http://jama.amaassn.org/cgi/content/full/294/3/351?ijkey=5f2cc4dad69d 6dc82c9fece1dec337cc75db60fc

29. *Take Control of your Health.* Dr. Joseph Mercola (2007).

30. National Research Council. Dietary Reference Intakes: *The Essential Guide to Nutrient Requirements. Washington, DC*: The National Academies Press, 2006.

31. Kimpimäki, T., Erkkola, M., Korhonen, S., Kupila, A., Virtanen, S. M., Ilonen, J., . . . Knip, M. (2001). *Short-term exclusive breastfeeding predisposes young children with increased genetic risk of type I diabetes to progressive beta-cell autoimmunity.* Diabetologia, 44(1), 63-9.

32. Phlips, J.C., Radermecker, R.P. *Type 1 diabetes: from genetic predisposition to hypothetical environmental triggers.* Rev Med Liege (Revue Medicale de Liege, Universite de Liege) Article in French. 2012 May-Jun;67(5-6):319-25. Retrieved from PubMed, http://www.ncbi.nlm.nih.gov/pubmed/22891485

231

33. Kant, Ashima. Consumption of energy-dense, nutrient-poor foods by adult Americant: nutritional and health inplications. The third National health and Nutrition Examination Survey, 1988-1994. Am J Clin Nutr October 2000.

34. Bray GA, Smith SR, de Jonge L, et al. *Effect of Dietary Protein Content on Weight Gain, Energy Expenditure, and Body Composition During Overeating: A Randomized Controlled Trial.* JAMA. 2012;307(1):47-55. doi:10.1001/jama.2011.1918.

35. *Dietary Intake of Protein Is Positively Associated with Percent Body Fat in Middle-Aged and Older Adults.* J. Nutr. March 1, 2011 141:440-446

36. Loenneke JP, Balapur A, Thrower AD, Syler G, Timlin M, Pujol TJ.. Ann Nutr Metab. 2010;57(3-4):219-20. Epub 2010 Dec 2. *Short report: Relationship between quality protein, lean mass and bone health.*

37. Halton TL, Hu FB. *The effects of high protein diets on thermogenesis, satiety and weight loss: a critical review.* J Am Coll Nutr. 2004 Oct;23(5):373-85.

38. The number 216,000 refers to the number of deaths caused by a form of cancer in the U.S. in <u>one single year</u>. The Civil War lasted from 1861-1865 and listed approximately 625,000 deaths over a 4 year period and World War II is noted as claiming the lives of over 405,000 Americans, however this number too reflects a total number of deaths over a 4 year period from 1941-1945.

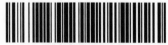
65442394R00151

Made in the USA
Middletown, DE
27 February 2018